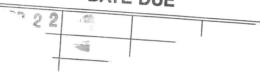

SPECIMEN DISSECTION
AND
PHOTOGRAPHY

SPECIMEN DISSECTION AND PHOTOGRAPHY

For the Pathologist, Anatomist and Biologist

By

M. DONALD McGAVIN, M.V.SC., PH.D., M.A.C.V.SC.

Diplomate of the American College of Veterinary Pathologists
Professor and Director of Laboratory Services
Department of Pathobiology
College of Veterinary Medicine
University of Tennessee
Knoxville, Tennessee

and

SAMUEL WESLEY THOMPSON, D.V.M., M.S.

Diplomate of the American College of Veterinary Pathologists
National Programs Director
of the Charles Louis Davis, D.V.M. Foundation
for the Advancement of Veterinary Pathology
Sayre, Pennsylvania
and
Consultant-Veterinary and Comparative Pathology

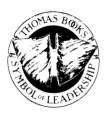

CHARLES C THOMAS · PUBLISHER
Springfield · Illinois · U.S.A.

Published and Distributed Throughout the World by

CHARLES C THOMAS • PUBLISHER
2600 South First Street
Springfield, Illinois 62717

© *1988 by* CHARLES C THOMAS • PUBLISHER

ISBN 0-398-05451-7

Library of Congress Catalog Card Number: 87-33676

With THOMAS BOOKS, *careful attention is given to all details of manufacturing
and design. It is the Publisher's desire to present books that are satisfactory as to their
physical qualities and artistic possibilities and appropriate for their particular use.*
THOMAS BOOKS *will be true to those laws of quality that assure a good name
and good will.*

Printed in the United States of America
SC-R-3

Library of Congress Cataloging-in-Publication Data

McGavin, M. Donald.
    Specimen dissection and photography : for the pathologist,
anatomist, and biologist / by M. Donald McGavin and Samuel Wesley
Thompson.
       p.   cm.
    Bibliography: p.
    Includes index.
    ISBN 0-398-05451-7
    1. Autopsy.   2. Human dissection.   3. Photography, Medical.
I. Thompson, Samuel Wesley. II. Title.
    [DNLM: 1. Dissection—methods.   2. Photography—methods.
3. Specimen Handling—methods.   QS 130 M478s]
RB27.M39   1988
778.9'9611—dc19
DNLM/DLC
for Library of Congress   87-33676
                                   CIP

PREFACE

Illustrations of pathological lesions and clinical conditions are an essential part in teaching medicine and biology. Numerous photographs are taken each year, but evaluation of transparencies projected in classrooms and at conferences reveal that many of them are not optimal. Obvious defects include poorly dissected lesions, anatomically incorrectly oriented specimens, obtrusive and messy backgrounds, inappropriate rulers and scales and poor photographic technique. The latter is usually because of flat lighting which provides no modeling. No doubt in many cases the poor photography is because of the lack of the services of a skilled biomedical photographer. However, poor specimen preparation is a more frequent limitation to a good photograph than the photographic technique—particularly in color transparencies.

Therefore, we have reviewed the literature and attempted to present a rational approach to the preparation and photography of specimens discussing the many variables involved—lighting, backgrounds, rulers, control of specular highlights and planning of facilities. In some cases there is no easy answer—a good example is the difficulty in obtaining a grey background of constant reflectance without color casts. Much can be done to improve the photography of specimens and animals by planning facilities and selecting equipment on the basis of rigid criteria—many of which are discussed in this text. Also, the introduction of new equipment, such as a camera with twin dedicated flash units, one acting as a modeling light and the other on reduced output as a fill-in light has greatly facilitated obtaining flash photographs with good modeling lighting. This is a major advance over the flat lighting from a single light source widely used in cadaver and clinical photography.

Unfortunately it is inevitable that despite great care there will be errors and omissions. We would appreciate colleagues drawing our attention to these in order to improve later editions.

ACKNOWLEDGMENT

In the preparation of this book, we have been fortunate in having received considerable assistance from colleagues who have shared designs and ideas and who have allowed us to reproduce illustrations from published works. All of the line diagrams, except those specifically acknowledged, were drawn by Ms. Linda J. LeFevre, B.S. (Medical Illustration), 6478 Ann Leigh Drive, North Rose, NY 14576. For additional illustrations we are also indebted to:

Mr. Max A. Robinson, School of Architecture, University of Tennessee for Figures 1.1 and 1.3.

University of Tennessee Photographic Services, Figure 1.4.

Bogen Photo Corporation, Figure 1.5.

Colortran, Inc., Figures 1.7 and 1.8.

Dr. L.J. LeBeau and the Editor, *Journal of Biological Photography* for Figures 1.9, 4.40 and 5.13.

Mr. H. Kreis Weigel for Figures 1.11, 2.11, 2.14 and 4.20.

Editor, *Medical and Biological Illustration,* Figure 2.3.

Department of Veterinary Pathology, Ontario Veterinary College, University of Guelph, Figures 2.6 and 2.7.

Dr. Ian Wilkie, Figure 2.7.

Editor, *British Journal of Photography,* Figure 2.8.

Mr. A. Smialosky and Dr. D.J. Curry, Figure 2.10 and 3.13.

Dr. Charle J. Burton, American Cyanamid Company and Editor, *Journal of Applied Physics,* and Drs. T.G. and E.G. Rochow for Figure 3.1.

Mr. A.F. Burry and Dr. B. Stewart and the Editor, *Medical and Biological Illustration,* Figure 3.9.

Editor, *Australian Veterinary Journal* for Figures 4.43, 4.44 and 4.45.

Dr. G.I. Alexander for Figure 5.3.

Dean, College of Veterinary Medicine, Kansas State University, Figure 5.5.

Dr. J.G. Morris for Figure 5.7.

Williams Photo Retouching, Knoxville, Tennessee for Figure 5.8.

We are grateful to Mr. David Blankenbeckler for retouching some figures.

Because many of the articles reviewed were scattered in a wide variety of journals, it was necessary to obtain these by interlibrary loan. We are particularly appreciative of the work by the librarians of the Agriculture-Veterinary Medicine Library of the University of Tennessee—Ms. Jean W. Taylor, Ms. Charlta B. Carter, and Ms. D. Marie Ruby.

We would like to express our sincere gratitude to Mrs. Jan Grady for her care, expertise, and dedication in typing the manuscript through its numerous drafts and to its final form. The senior author would also like to express his gratitude to the instructors of the Central Technical College, Brisbane, Australia, to Mr. Ernie Hollywood, formerly Chief Medical Photographer, University of Queensland Medical School, Brisbane, Australia and to Mr. C.G. Spiers for their advise. Finally, we would like to recognize the support and understanding of our wives during the preparation of this manuscript.

CONTENTS

SPECIMEN DISSECTION
AND
PHOTOGRAPHY

Chapter 1

FACILITIES AND EQUIPMENT

The photographic industry is burgeoning. New versatile equipment appears rapidly and thus recommendations of specific models are often soon out of date. It is more important for the reader to understand the criteria for choosing equipment rather than to know brand names and model numbers. Items unavailable commercially or, if available, inadequate in performance will have to be custom made. If all the equipment needed was commercially available, there would be little need to list criteria and discuss deficiencies in equipment, such as photographic stands and transilluminated backgrounds.

NECROPSY PHOTOGRAPHY ROOM

It is common practice in many hospitals to photograph pathological specimens in the same studio and with the same equipment and backgrounds used for routine photography. This practice cannot be too strongly condemned because of the danger of contamination of equipment with pathogenic microorganisms and the resultant spread of infection. This has been shown by LeBeau (1973) who recovered *Staphylococcus aureus* from the cable release and focusing ring of a camera and the glass specimen plate after photography of lungs with a staphylococcal pneumonia.

Numerous authors (Stanford, 1946; Martin, 1961; Burgess, 1975) have recommended a separate room with separate equipment for autopsy specimen photography. Equipment may become contaminated by infectious organisms and thus should not be removed from the necropsy area (Fritts, 1976). A small locked room where equipment can be stored safely but ready for immediate use expedites photography. The exact location of this room in relation to the necropsy room has been debated. Martin (1961) recommends that it be near the darkroom, but the obvious place to reduce the possibility of spread of infection is immediately next to the necropsy room. Opinion varies as to whether access should be only from the necropsy room or whether the room should have two entrances, one from a "clean" corridor and the other from the necropsy room itself. The latter arrangement can provide an unauthorized entrance to the necropsy room. For this reason, our photography room has only one entrance: from the necropsy room itself (Fig. 1.1). This means that only necropsy personnel, correctly garbed, have access to it when the necropsy room is in use. However, after cleaning, outside personnel can enter. Obviously, the room should be secluded so the public does not have ready access to it.

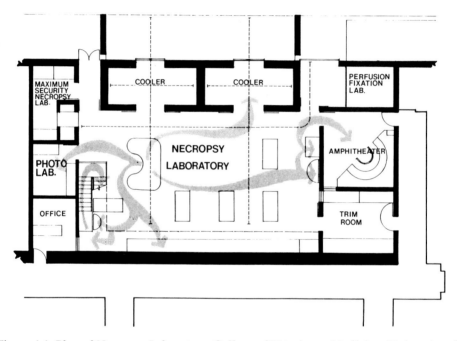

Figure 1.1. Plan of Necropsy Laboratory, College of Veterinary Medicine, University of Tennessee. The Photography Room is close to the autopsy tables.

Rather than a separate photographic room, some veterinary necropsy laboratories have an alcove or space in the necropsy room itself (Fritts, 1976). These are not as desirable as a separate room. Photographic equipment cannot be locked away conveniently and film and equipment can be damaged by high humidity from water or steam used to clean the necropsy room. Other veterinary necropsy facilities have the photographic room adjacent to the laboratory but on the "clean" side of the entrance to the necropsy facility. This is inappropriate, because the specimen should always be regarded as contaminated and potentially dangerous. It is very convenient if the photography room is adjacent to the "trim" room (Fig. 1.1)—the room in which fixed tissues and surgical biopsies are trimmed prior to processing to histological sections. Brains are routinely fixed for days or weeks before being sliced, and cross sections of brain frequently need to be photographed. Also, large unfixed surgical specimens received at the trim room may need to be photographed, emphasizing the desirability of the photography room being adjacent to the trim room. If the arrangement of the necropsy room and the trim room is such that one photography room cannot be shared, an alternative arrangement is to have two photography rooms or areas—one for necropsy specimens and the other for fixed and therefore non-infectious tissues. If the trim room is large, photographic equipment can be housed in one corner, although a separate lockable room is desirable.

ROOM DESIGN

As the room is used to dissect and prepare specimens for photography, it should contain all the necessary equipment and supplies. It should also have an efficient labor-saving design to minimize wasteful movements. Engel (1961) points out that too large a room results in inefficiency and excess walking. Good design makes it easy to maintain "clean" and "dirty" areas and expedite cleaning. Stanford (1946) and Gibson (1948) both recommend a 10 × 8 ft. studio. Gibson (1948) recommends that the preparation of specimens take place in a 3 × 4 ft. alcove adjacent to an 8 × 10 ft. studio. This recommendation is based on the assumption that all "dirty" work will be done in the alcove, and that only "clean" work will be done in the studio. In fact, backgrounds need to be cleaned, specimens propped up or trimmed, and hands and gloves washed frequently while the specimen is still under the camera. Thus, it is highly desirable to have, in the studio, both clean and dirty areas with sinks.

In our experience, a room 11 × 10 ft. (Fig. 1.2) is barely adequate, as it does not allow sufficient room to move the fill-in lamp to provide a 3:1 (much less a 4:1) lighting ratio sometimes desired for monochrome photography. A 14 × 10 ft. room is required, reserving the 14 ft. side for the vertically mounted camera and its lamps. The photography room of the Pathology Department, Ontario Veterinary College, University of Guelph, is 14 ft. long which is sufficient to allow the use of a 4 × 2-½ ft. transilluminated light box (Fig. 2.6). Our room, with an 11 ft. side, barely accommodates a 2-½ ft. wide box. Although a 14 ft. long room is highly desirable, the room should be no wider than 10 or 11 ft. so that the distance from the camera to the stainless steel specimen counter and sink is convenient (Fig. 1.2)..The door opening should be 32 to 36 inches wide to allow easy ingress of 48 × 30 inches background boards on which animal cadavers weighing up to 70 lb. weight are carried. It is advantageous for the photographer to be able to see what is going on in the necropsy room. If the door is not suitably placed, a small window should be inserted in the wall or door. Walls should be white, semigloss and easy to clean. Epoxy-painted masonry blocks are satisfactory. The ceiling should also be impervious and resistant to moisture and painted flat black to prevent reflections in glass-topped specimen boxes. Fluorescent lamps are used to provide a high level of illumination for room cleaning and specimen dissection. During photography, room light is provided by several incandescent lamps located over the specimen-preparation counter (Fig. 1.2), where they cannot reflect light off the glass-topped specimen box into the camera. These lamps provide adequate illumination for focusing and framing, but because their level of illumination is relatively low compared to that of the photographic lamps, and because they do not reflect in the glass supporting the specimen, they do not have to be turned off during actual photography, a real convenience.

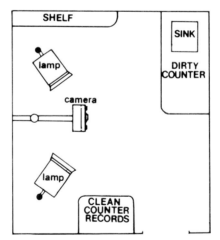

Figure 1.2. Plan of Necropsy Photography Room to show the "clean" and "dirty" areas. The room is 10 × 11 feet, but a room 10 × 14 feet is more desirable to allow flexibility in positioning lights.

To prevent contamination of equipment, "clean" and "dirty" areas must be clearly marked. In ours, the "dirty" areas are a sink, a stainless steel dissection counter with a 1 inch lip, background boards and the specimen support glasses on the black and light boxes. A small "clean" counter holds the record books and extra photographic equipment (Fig. 1.2). The cabinets over this counter are also "clean." The large sink at the end of the stainless steel counter is used for washing background boards and glasses from specimen background boxes. The sink has a swivelling goosenecked faucet fitted with an aerator and a knee-operated valve. Paper towel and soap dispensers are mounted close to the sink. Neutral buffered 10% formalin (NBF) and Jores' solutions are piped to the sink from reservoirs outside of the room. Dissection equipment, long straight bladed knives, retractors and disposable gloves are kept in a drawer under the "dirty" counter. A small ledge holds the vertically placed background boards just above the floor so that the floor can be cleaned easily and boards can drain and dry. There is a small open "dirty" shelf to hold background props, black wooden blocks, modeling clay, rulers and glass cleaner (Fig. 1.2). An open shelf is preferred to a cabinet, as doors do not have to be opened.

Climate Control

The temperature, humidity and air exchanges per hour must be controlled. Excess heat and low humidity cause specimens to dry out, and sufficient air changes are recommended to remove formalin fumes and the smell of some specimens. Our room is maintained at 66°F to 68°F, 40% to 50% relative humidity and it has 10 air changes per hour. The direction of air flow is extremely important to control odors and reduce aerosol infections. Williams (1984) raises the possibility of aerosol infection being caused by infectious exudates and specimens being dried out by the warm photographic lights. The air flow should carry microorganisms and odors away from the operator. To do this, air should enter through grills in or near the ceiling and exit through ducts mounted a few inches above floor level (Fig. 1.3).

Floor

Because blood and exudates drop onto the floor, this must be impervious and designed so that it can be hosed clean easily. Concrete is suitable, but to prevent the formation of dust it must be sealed with light grey epoxy paint or a surface such as Stonhard®. The floor should slope

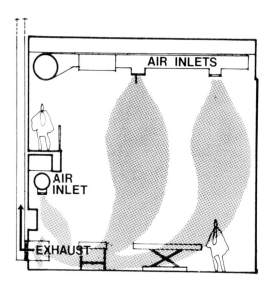

Figure 1.3. Side elevation of Necropsy Laboratory to show the down-draft ventilation which minimizes odors and carries pathogenic organisms and toxic fumes away from the operator's face.

to a drain or drains, but unless the floor under the camera is flat, background boxes mounted on castors will be unstable. Castors of adjustable height are essential to compensate for irregularities in the floor. Contractors are frequently not successful in meeting specifications on sloping floors, and it is not unusual that the highest point in the room is the drain. In a photography room the floor should have the following features:

1. **Slope.** The floor should be flat over at least a 6 ft. × 3 ft. area centered under the camera so that the background boxes will be horizontal and all 4 of their castors will be in contact with the floor. The remainder of the floor or even the whole floor should slope uniformly towards the wall behind the photographic stand so that spills flow away from the operator. A fall of 1 inch in 6 to 8 ft. is adequate. Castors on the background boxes should be adjustable so that the box can be adjusted to be horizontal. The worst floor is one which slopes at varying degrees to a central drain, as castors cannot be adjusted to ensure that all four wheels are in contact with all portions of the floor.

2. **Color.** Colored walls should be avoided, as they may cause color casts by reflecting light onto the specimen. Thus, walls should be white or a neutral light grey. White walls can be used to reflect light as fill-in

illumination. A light grey epoxy painted floor can be used as a background for very large organs. Some floors are covered by light grey vinyl, but this is not as sanitary as epoxy paint.

A hose with a mixing faucet of hot and cold water should be available to wash down the floor. The only items on the floor should be the background boxes and lamp tripods. The latter are aluminum to prevent rust. The boxes on castors can be moved while the floor is hosed and squeegeed. Excessively hot water and steam should be avoided, as the resultant high humidity may damage equipment.

Recommendations. A lockable separate photographic room should be located immediately adjacent to the necropsy room. To allow flexibility in the positioning of lights, its dimensions should not be less than 14 × 10 ft. The design in Figure 1.2 is good. The floor should be light grey, the walls white and the ceiling black. Clean and dirty areas should be clearly defined (Fig. 1.2). Ceiling lights should be positioned over the preparation bench so that they do not reflect into the camera off the glass of the specimen box. Thus, they can be left on during photography.

EQUIPMENT

Photostand

Nowadays, photographs of gross specimens are taken by a vertically mounted camera (Fig. 1.4). Originally, cameras were mounted on tripods (Levin, 1939), but these were cumbersome to use and the legs of the camera tripod and the lamp tripods were easily bumped out of position. The vertically mounted camera has the advantages that the specimen does not have to be pinned to the background and specimens can be photographed immersed under fluid. Also, the vertical camera angle excludes excess background (Clarke, 1933), and interchanging opaque and transilluminated light backgrounds is easy. The use of vertically mounted camera stands is not new. Martinsen (1952) in his review cites Ward (1902) and Schmidt and Haulenbeek (1932) who fabricated stands. Clarke (1933) and Martinsen (1952) recommend the use of an "old style x-ray tube stand which is adjustable to any tilt angle." A different model of x-ray tube stand which allowed the camera to be moved from left to right (Y-axis) or swivelled on the camera's optical axis (i.e. on the X-axis) was modified by Wolfe (1983). The recommendations to use a modified x-ray tube stand are an indication that many of the commercially available models lack versatility, particularly for use with large specimens. This is not surprising, because the majority of the commercial stands are designed for copying flat artwork.

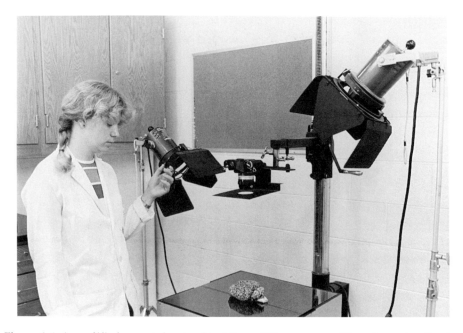

Figure 1.4. A modified x-ray tube stand holding a Nikon camera. Note the anti-reflection shield under the camera's lens. The camera and the brain are incorrectly oriented anatomically. A vertical format should be used in a dorsal view of whole brain.

Therefore, to select a stand, it is necessary for the reader to have an appreciation for desirable features. The versatility of the equipment greatly affects the speed and ease of photography of gross specimens. Time taken for photography of gross specimens should be kept to a minimum for the following reasons:

1. Specimens dry out and lose "bloom" because of dehydration; for example, fresh fibrinous exudates become amorphous and lose fine fibrillar structure after 5 to 10 minutes, even if not exposed to studio lights.
2. Congested specimens may ooze blood from their edges and thus there is a continual battle to keep the background clean.
3. Infectious material is potentially dangerous, and time of exposure to it should be reduced to a minimum.

4. Delay in fixation. For optimum histopathological and electron microscopic examinations, tissues must be fixed with minimum delay after death.

Desirable Features in a Stand

These have been discussed (McGavin, 1982). The stand should allow the camera to be adjusted in the following directions:

1. Vertically to frame and focus.
2. X- and Y-axis, i.e. X = towards and away from the front of the column.
   Y = to left and right of the column.
3. Change from vertical to horizontal format.
4. Rotate on the X-axis to allow camera to focus on planes not at 90° to the vertical column.

All of these features except number 4 are present in the Bogen Maxi Repro Stand® (Fig. 1.5) made by IFF, Firenza, Italy.

1. **Positioning of the Column.** It is generally desirable to fasten the vertical column directly to the wall. Most commercial stands are sold as copy stands, and wall mounting brackets may or may not be available. Thus, frequently custom-made brackets are needed. As it is critical that the column be exactly vertical, brackets should be designed so that minor adjustments can be made to achieve this vertical position. The question which arises is how far from the wall should the brackets extend to hold the column? This distance, which should be kept to a minimum to reduce vibration, needs to be sufficient to allow the handle of the rack and pinion to rotate and allow the adjustable X-arm (see below) to be moved in and out. Another advantage of having the column mounted on a reasonably long bracket is that lights can be placed on either side of the column to illuminate cavities. One way to minimize the length of the brackets and thus vibration and yet have sufficient room to place lights is to mount the column by short brackets onto a central pillar which then has clearance on both sides (Fig. 1.6). Even a pillar which protrudes from the wall by 1-1/2 to 2 feet (Fig. 1.6) is an advantage.

Clarke (1933) describes a camera stand that avoided these difficulties and had the advantage of keeping a large clear floor space for specimens or lighting. The camera was supported on a vertically mounted 2-1/2 × 4 in. I beam held rigidly and perpendicular to the ceiling by three 1/4 in. iron guy rods fastened to the walls near the ceiling. The vertical movement of the camera was counterbalanced. This design had advantages. It

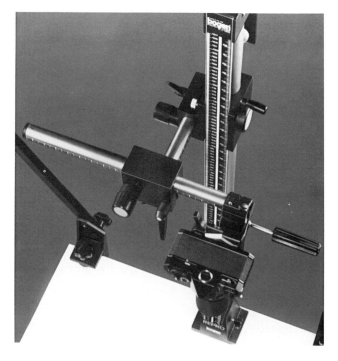

Figure 1.5. Bogen Maxi-Repro Stand®. The camera can be moved from left to right and towards and away from the stand. A stand of this type has replaced the stand depicted in Figure 1.4.

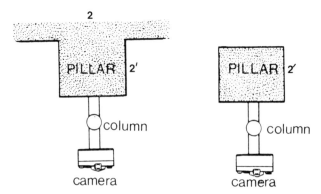

Figure 1.6. A wall-mounted stand attached to a pillar has the advantage of having more space to allow photographic lamps to be positioned at the top of the frame, thus increasing the flexibility of the lighting.

allowed maximum flexibility of positioning lights and a maximum specimen area. Also, a rigidly mounted I beam was less prone to vibrate than
a column mounted by long brackets to a wall. The length of the X arm,
the one extending towards the operator, did not limit the size of the
specimen, as the specimen box could be pushed under the stand supports.
To photograph very large specimens, the X arm still needed to be
sufficiently long to allow the camera's field of view to clear the end of the
I beam. To allow extreme close-ups such as at a ratio of reproduction
(RR) of 1:1 (life-size), with a 50mm lens on a 35mm camera, the lower end
of the I beam would have to extend within approximately 6 inches of the
specimen.

The position of the lower end of the wall-mounted column should be
decided by the lowest working position of the camera, e.g. when the
camera is focused on a specimen at RR = 1:1. For most 50mm lenses on a
35mm camera this will be 4 inches from the nodal point. A more practical way to handle this is to mount the stand so when the camera is at its
lowest position, the front edge of the 50mm lens is 3 inches but no closer
to the top of the specimen background. This will ensure that the camera
can be lowered sufficiently to obtain an RR = 1:1 when the specimen is
placed directly on the background but will prevent the camera from
hitting the background. Obviously, to make this decision the height of
the background must be selected. By trial and error we have found that a
28-inch high background is suitable for specimens varying from 3 to 20
inches in length (Fig. 2.6). This height allows the photographer to lean
over comfortably to focus the camera on most specimens. If only very
small specimens are to be photographed, a higher background would be
desirable to reduce bending and thus fatigue in the photographer. Large
commercial copy stands usually have built-in tables which are 20 to 26
inches in height. The table height should be selected on the basis of a
comfortable working position for the photographer. This will depend
upon the size of the specimens and the focal length and thus the working
distance of the lens used. Because the table height is a compromise, it is
best decided by trial and error with specimens of various sizes and with
lenses of different focal lengths.

Another critical feature is rigidity. Clarke (1933) recommends that to
reduce the effects of vibration, the camera and specimen supports should
be separate (Fig. 1.4). It is essential that there be no vibration in the walls,
for example, from heavy machinery or that the brackets be so flimsy that
manipulation of the camera sets up a vibration in them. Similarly, the X

arm which protrudes horizontally from the column towards the operator must also not vibrate after such manipulations as cocking the shutter. Minor vibration is inevitable, and thus it is necessary to delay exposures for several seconds after touching the camera or alternatively to use electronic flash. The stand needs to be so well machined that there is little backlash or slack so that framing is not changed as the camera is manipulated. Wear in the rack-and-pinion drive can result in a significant side-to-side movement of the X arm. Even a ¼ inch side movement of the camera will result in incorrect framing and, for example, the ruler may be partially obscured.

2. **Vertical Adjustment.** This is usually rack-and-pinion, counterbalanced or friction drive (Figs. 1.4 and 1.5). Counterbalanced units have the disadvantage that the correct counterbalance for one camera may be too light or too heavy for another. For preciseness and ease of adjustment, rack-and-pinion drives have no peer, although they do tend to wear and develop slack. The length of the vertical column dictates the maximum size of field that can be framed. Thus, with small animals a short column such as that on a table-mounted copy stand is adequate, but specimens from large animals require a column with approximately 48 inches of useful vertical camera movement. Commercially available stands have columns that vary from 42 to 57 inches in height, and some floor-mounted models are 88 inches in height.

3. **X and Y Adjustments.** The X-axis or arm is at 90° to the column and extends towards the operator. The Y-axis is to the left and right of the column at right angles to the X-axis (Fig. 1.5). These types of adjustment are not available on all copy stands, and in those cases, there is no alternative but to move the background, e.g. a small black box on rollers (Vetter, 1969) or large background boxes on castors. Disadvantages in moving the background are:

1. Delicately balanced specimens, props and rulers may fall as the background is moved.
2. If the floor is not level, the plane of the specimen may not be parallel to the film plane. Also, if the floor is not flat the box may be moved to a position where it is unstable because all four feet or castors are not in contact with the floor.
3. Infectious material. If the box does not have to be moved, there is no chance of the photographer touching infectious material.

The X arm should be long enough to extend over the center of the background box and also allow some clearance between the box and the column. To reach the center of a 21 × 21 inch box, the X arm needs to be 10 to 15 inches long, measured from column to the optical center of the lens. Most commercial stands do not have an X arm as long as this. If the X arm is relatively short, it simply means that the whole surface of the background cannot be used and the camera cannot photograph large specimens.

4. **Rotation of Camera on X Arm Around its Long Axis.** This feature is present in some commercial stands and is desirable for close-up photography of subjects where their surface is in a plane not parallel to the plane of the background. A good example is a brain. Rotation of the camera allows a better viewing angle and also places the camera's film plane parallel to the plane of the surface of the specimen, thus reducing the need for a large depth of field to have the whole specimen in focus. In fact, with small brains photographed at an RR = 1:3, the depth of field of 18mm at f-22 is not adequate to bring the whole brain into focus, and the only alternative is not to fill the frame with the image of the subject but to use an RR of 1:5 or 1:6 to obtain adequate depth of field and thus have the whole of the subject in focus. Occasionally, the background has to be tilted to allow the light of the fixed lamps to illuminate the specimen optimally. Thus, the ability to rotate the camera so that its film plane is still parallel to the plane of the specimen is an advantage.

5. **Change from Horizontal to Vertical Format.** The ability to change the camera from horizontal to vertical format without significant change in the position of its optical axis is highly desirable. Specimens should always be placed in their anatomically correct position and then framed in the viewfinder. Thus, long bones should be vertical and a vertical camera format used. Ease of changing from horizontal to vertical formats encourages the use of correct anatomical orientation. With standardized lighting, lamps are positioned at fixed distances from the subject and the correct exposure determined for a horizontal format. If a change to a vertical format moves the camera's optical axis several inches to the side, the subject will have to be moved closer to one lamp, thus requiring a change in exposure, particularly if only one lamp is used. A moveable bracket, the Vertaflip® (The Saunders Group, 67 Deep Rock Road, Rochester, N.Y. 14624) solves this problem, as it allows the camera to be changed from a horizontal to a vertical format without significant change in the position of the camera's optical axis. However, this device

was designed to support a small electronic flash unit and to change its position when a camera was changed from a vertical to a horizontal format. Any vibration was eliminated by the short duration of the flash exposure. When the Vertaflip is used with a heavy camera in a horizontal position on a copy stand, vibrations can be introduced. An alternative method of supporting the camera is to have either a swiveling bracket or to have two camera attachment devices (see 7 below), one for the horizontal and the other for the vertical format. However, changing the camera from one bracket to the other will result in a change in the position of the optical axis, and thus either the specimen or the camera will have to be repositioned. The Vertaflip which avoids this problem of change in optical axis can be used but with electronic flash illumination to neutralize the effects of vibration.

6. **Camera Leveling on Side Arm.** Bencher (333 W. Lake St., Chicago, Illinois 60606) markets a "precision camera leveling plate" which can be adjusted to compensate for lack of any parallelism between the film and camera planes. This can be caused by the weight of a heavy camera depressing the X arm or by an uneven floor tilting the background box.

7. **Camera Attachment Devices.** Bencher and Bogen market quick-release devices which allow easy removal of a camera to facilitate reloading and yet retain the camera's position when it is remounted. This feature really expedites reloading of cameras. Some stands, particularly custom-made stands, use a ball-and-socket head mounted at the end of the side arm. These are contraindicated for several reasons. The major one is that they do not incorporate any mechanism to maintain parallelism between the film and specimen planes, and checking this is easily forgotten at the time when the camera is replaced after reloading. Also, some ball-and-socket heads can slowly drift out of position. The camera's film plane should be carefully checked for parallelism with the specimen plane by using a bull's-eye bubble placed on the back of the camera. This check should be done at least every time the camera is remounted, usually after reloading, unless a precentered quick-release device is used. Failure to maintain parallelism results in distortion known as "keystoning" in which a rectangle is recorded as a trapezoid with one pair of sides converging.

8. **Control of Reflections of the Camera and Stand in a Glass-Covered Background Box.** Such reflections are inevitable, and to control them,

the ceiling, camera-stand and brackets should all be painted a non-reflective dull matte black. Unfortunately, some finely engineered photographic stands are either gleaming stainless or chromium-plated steel. However, complete prevention requires the use of a reflection control shield such as a black card or a black metal sheet below the camera lens. Unfortunately, the size of the card necessary to shield the whole of the field of view depends on the size of the field of view of the camera. Thus, large specimens need large shields and small ones, small shields. A large one cannot be used for all specimens, because as the camera moves closer to the specimen and the RR approaches 1:2, the large shield obstructs light from the lamps falling on the subject. Thus, a smaller shield has to be used. Also, it is difficult to position the shield correctly by mounting it on the stand below the camera. The lens mount may or may not be in the middle of the camera body, and the physical length of lenses vary. To overcome these difficulties, commercial shields are now manufactured which screw directly into the lens filter mount. However the most convenient position for the shield is an inch or two below the lens rim. This allows sufficient room for the operator's hand to reach the focusing ring. However, it is difficult to mount shields this way so that both 55mm and 105mm macro-lenses and different camera bodies can be used.

Commercial stands are available from Bencher (333 W. Lake St., Chicago, Illinois 60606), Bogen (Bogen Photo Corp., Fair Lawn, NJ 07410), Linhof (H.P. Marketing Corp., Linhof Division, 216 Little Falls Rd., Cedar Grove, NJ 07009), and Polaroid (Polaroid Corp., 549 Technology Square, Cambridge, Mass. 02139). Columns range in heights from 42 to 57 inches, and movement on the X-axis varies from 0 to 11 inches. Designs are changing constantly and models need to be evaluated carefully for the suitability of their features. At the time of writing, no commercial stand offers all of the features described above, but the Bogen Maxi-Repro Stand has most of these (Fig. 1.5). It has 46 inches of usable column and side arms that can move in and out and left to right for approximately 13 inches, and the format is easily changed from horizontal to vertical. With this unit, the camera is normally mounted on the right end of the arm that moves from side to side (Fig. 1.5). This causes no difficulty when used with copying lights, but with the main light to the left and slightly above (Fig. 3.7), the arm casts a shadow on the subject. Therefore, the camera should be mounted on the left end of the side-to-side arm. Minor changes by a machine shop are necessary to allow the camera to rotate from a horizontal to a vertical format. If only small specimens are photographed, then a bench top "copying stand" will be adequate.

Photographic Lamps

These are used to illuminate pathological specimens usually photographed by a camera mounted on a vertical stand. Selection of photographic lamps is critical to the success of photography of gross specimens, particularly in the flexibility of lighting (diffuse or flood vs. collimated or "hard") and the control of the size and number of specular highlights. Many laboratories use diffuse lighting, usually with 2 or 4 photoflood lamps in non-focusable reflectors. For a little more money, focusable flood-spot lamps could be purchased. Lamps should be selected on the basis of the size of their fields of illumination, flood or spot lighting, evenness of illumination and intensity of illumination. The latter category is critical, as this decides whether slow films which have the highest resolving power, lowest granularity value and often the highest saturation of colors can be used (see "Film"). In other words, lamps should be chosen to suit the film, not vice versa. Selection of lamps is usually a compromise among the following factors:

1. **Light Output, Usually 500–650 Watts.** The intensity of the illumination and the sensitivity of the film determines the exposure. Different models of photographic lamps have different light outputs. The lamp selected needs to have sufficient light output to allow an exposure with a lens aperture between f-16 and f-22 to obtain adequate depth of field and a shutter speed not slower than $1/8$ second. Shutter speeds slower than this will produce reciprocity failure with many films (Kodak, 1983). This subject is discussed under "Exposure."

2. **Heat Production.** Unfortunately, increased light output is accompanied by increased heat production which tends to damage and dry out specimens. Therefore, if 650W bulbs give adequate light, there is no point in using 1000W bulbs.

3. **Color Temperature.** It is essential that lamps accept bulbs whose rated color temperature matches the color temperature of the film. $3,200°K$ bulbs are available for most lamps, but $3400°K$ bulbs, which are necessary for type A color film such as Kodachrome 40, may not be

available. In that case, one alternative is to use 3,200°K bulbs with a light-balancing filter fitted either to the lamp or to the camera. The image in the viewfinder is colored which interferes with the photographer's ability to evaluate the image.

4. **Size of Illuminated Field.** Manufacturers state the beam diameter at specified distances (Figs. 1.7 and 1.8). The illuminated field size of the lamp should match the size of the specimen. If the largest specimen is 2 ft. in diameter, there is no advantage, but many disadvantages in selecting a lamp that will produce a 6 ft. diameter circle of illumination at the proposed lamp-subject distance.

5. **Collimation of Light.** Different model lamps vary in their ability to focus light into a parallel beam. The more parallel the beam, the "harder" the beam and the more sharply delineated the shadows. High-quality spotlamps often utilize a Fresnel lens to help focus light rays (Fig. 1.8). This adds to the cost and weight of the lamp and the instability of the stand. Because the Fresnel lens reduces air flow and cooling, some of these spotlamps have blowers, further adding to the weight and cost. Lamps without Fresnel lenses produce a relatively parallel beam adequate for most large specimens. For extremely small specimens such as those from laboratory animals, small changes in modeling must be accentuated and a parallel beam is essential.

6. **Flood-Spot Focusing Lamps.** We selected lamps with this feature because they can be adjusted from a hard modeling or texture light to a diffuse fill-in light. Different models of focusing spotlamps vary in their ability to produce even illumination at different settings of the flood-to-spot adjustment. This should always be checked by a spot meter or trial exposures with the circle of illumination required.

7. **Diameter of the Reflector.** The size of specular highlights is directly proportional to the size of the light source. Therefore, the smaller the diameter of the reflector capable of giving the desired circle of even illumination, the better.

8. **Weight.** In a fixed lighting arrangement, lamps do not have to be moved and weight is of little importance except for its effect on the stability of lamp stands.

9. **Stability of Stands.** Many lamps and stands are sold separately. A stand must be selected for stability. The heavier the lamp, the more robust the stand must be, and the wider the spread of the tripod legs of the stand required. This latter feature can be a problem. Widely spaced

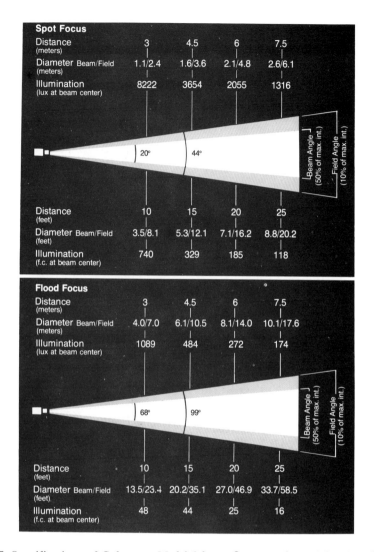

Figure 1.7. Specifications of Colortran Multi-6 lamps® at spot-focus (*above*) and flood-focus (*below*). The beam increases in diameter from 3½ to 13½ feet from spot to flood.

tripod legs prevent the lateral movement of the light box (Fig. 1.4) and impinge on the specimen area. Because floors have to be washed frequently, stands should be non-rusting, e.g. aluminum.

10. **Accessories: Polarizing Filters, Diffusers, Barn Doors.** The availability, cost and ease of attachment of these need to be checked. Barn doors— metal flaps hinged on the rims of the lamp (Fig. 1.4)—are helpful in shielding light from the operator's face and allow him to focus and

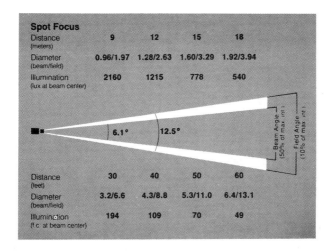

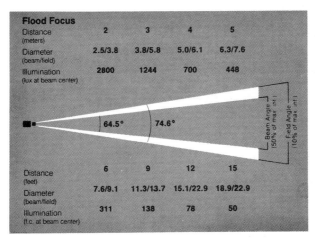

Figure 1.8. Specifications of a Colortran 6 inch Theatre Fresnel®.

compose without the distraction of glaring light or heat. Polarizing filters are costly and easily damaged. Because they are not required for most specimens, polarizers need not be in place permanently and their ease of attachment and removal is important. Also, some polarizing filters are damaged by high-intensity light and heat, and a high/low light output switch for the lamps may be required. These are available for some, but not all, modern halogen lamps. If only 3,200°K lamps are available, then to use a type A film such as Kodachrome 40, a light-balancing filter will be needed to raise the color temperature to 3,400°K. The availability of filter holders to fit the lamps should be checked.

11. **Cost.** Lamps are not cheap and the ultimate choice will probably be a compromise. However, the range in price is considerable, and lamps suitable for most specimens are available at modest cost. Because lamp houses and stands are sold separately, only the lamp house will need to be replaced if a better model is acquired.

12. **Number.** This was discussed under "Lighting." Two lamps are minimal, a modeling lamp to be placed at 60° from the camera-subject axis and a similar lamp as a "fill-in" at 45° (Fig. 3.6). However, photography is expedited if a "texture" lamp (with its axis at 75°–80° to the camera-subject axis) (Fig. 3.5) is mounted under the "modeling" lamp. This obviates the need to lower the "modeling" lamp to obtain "texture" lighting and, apart from saving time, has the advantage that a lamp need not be moved from its standardized angle, thus reducing a variable in photography.

Our equipment includes two photographic lamps mounted on tripod stands. They are fitted with 650W 3,400°K halogen bulbs and are focusable from flood to spot. The equipment supplied by Colortran Inc. (1015 Chestnut St., Burbank, California 91506) consists of:

> 2—Catalog # 100-151 Multi-6 lamps
> 2—Catalog # 118-013 4 leaf barn doors
> 2—Catalog # FCA 650W 3,400° K bulbs
> 1—Catalog # 152-003 Stand
> 1—Catalog # 152-019 Stand

The Multi-6 was designed for use at long distances in a theater. When used at a distance of 3-1/2 ft. from the subject, these lamps have a beam diameter of about 15 inches in the "spot" position and double that when the filament is positioned midway between "spot" and "flood." In the latter position, the illuminated area is adequate in size and evenness for most specimens. However, small movements of the "spot-flood" lever may result in unevenness of illumination and this should be checked carefully with a meter. Before ordering stands, it is desirable to check that they can be adjusted to the heights required, as for example in Figure 3.6. The Colortran Theatre Fresnel 6 (Fig. 1.8) incorporates a Fresnel lens which gives a narrower, more evenly illuminated beam. Comparison of the beam characteristics of the Multi-6 and the Theatre Fresnel 6 are given in Figures 1.7 and 1.8. The Theatre Fresnel 6 is a much larger and heavier lamp than the Multi-6 and too large to fit in our

11 ft. × 10 ft. photography room. The Multi-6 produces excellent results with most specimens from RR's from 1:12 to 1:2.

Electronic Flash Units

Electronic flash units are used for two main purposes: (1) as a substitute for photolamps to illuminate pathological specimens on a background box (Fig. 2.7); and (2) as a mobile source of illumination for clinical and cadaver photography.

The flash units for these two purposes have different requirements.

1. **Flash Unit for Pathological Specimens Under a Camera on a Vertical Photostand.** Haber (1982) used 4 flash heads, two pairs on each side of the specimen mounted at a 45° angle. To reduce specimen highlights, all flash heads were fitted with polarizing filters. Only one flash head was connected to the camera by a synchronizer cable. The other flash unit on the same side was "ganged" to it and the flash units on the other side were slave activated.

A different approach has been taken at the Ontario Veterinary College, University of Guelph. A single-flash head is mounted on each side of the specimen (Fig. 2.7). The unit has the following features. A modeling light is incorporated in the flash head so that the effect of the lighting can be evaluated visually. Power can be reduced to ¾, ½ or ¼ for each unit, thus allowing the amount of light to be controlled so that one lamp, usually the right, can be used as a fill-in light. If the flash unit does not allow reduction of output from an individual lamp, its light output can be reduced by the use of neutral density filters over the flash head as described by LeBeau (1985). Light output is sufficient to allow the use of apertures of f-11 to f-22 with 200 ISO film in order to obtain adequate depth of field.

This type of arrangement has the advantage of eliminating the effect of vibration, producing constant light output and allowing exposure standardization. A disadvantage is that the flash heads available cannot produce a parallel beam of light to produce well-delineated shadows (hard light) to emphasize surface texture. However, in a room where vibration from heavy equipment is a problem, electronic flash should be strongly considered.

2. **Cadaver and Clinical Photography.** Flash units have been used for this type of photography for decades, but there have, until recently, been marked difficulties in obtaining texture lighting with the correct

amount of fill-in illumination. The usual procedure was to place the flash unit near the camera, but this resulted in flat lighting with little indication of modeling or texture. Originally, all exposures had to be calculated from a so-called guide number which was based on the mathematical formula f = guide #/distance. Allowances had to be then estimated for reflections of light from walls and the reflectivity of the subject. Later, flash meters were developed and this was followed by automatic exposure devices for flash units with the sensor built into the unit itself. Later came remote sensors which could be mounted on the camera while the flash head was moved away to provide modeling illumination. The latest development is "dedicated" flash units whose light output and thus exposure is controlled by cells reading the light passing through the lens (TTL) and in some cases off the film (OTF). Although this gives excellent exposure control, many of these flash units could only be mounted directly onto the camera's "hot shoe" resulting in flat lighting. Recently, a synchronizing cord (DUO–SYN®, Altrex 7500 Skokie Blvd, Skokie, IL 60077) that connects the shoe of the dedicated flash unit to the camera's hot shoe has been marketed. This allows the flash head to be moved 4–6 ft. away from the camera to provide modeling illumination. Also, two of these synchronizer cords can be mated together to fire two flash units simultaneously. The advantage of this is that exposure of both flash units can be controlled by the TTL–OTF meters in the camera. Some flash units have variable power outputs and can be switched to a $\frac{1}{2}$, $\frac{1}{4}$ or $\frac{1}{8}$. Thus, one flash unit on full power can be held at 30°–45° to the subject to act as a modeling light and a second flash unit, mounted on the camera's hot shoe at $\frac{1}{4}$ output, provides the fill-in illumination. The camera, two flash units, and a handgrip are lightweight, self-contained and easy to use in a clinical examination room or in the contaminated environment of a necropsy room. The combination of two dedicated flash units fitted to a camera with TTL–OTF metering is a major advance in clinical and cadaver photography. Not only has the camera been easy to use, but photographs have had excellent modeling, both in monochrome and in color, and exposure control for average subjects has been highly reliable. Compensation must be made for very dark and very large subjects, as these mislead the meters. Further details on the use of dedicated units is described under "Cadaver, Photography and Clinical Photography."

Dedicated cameras and flash units are more expensive but are well worth the additional cost for clinical and cadaver photography. Currently, we are using a Pentax Super Program camera with two Pentax AF 200T flash units connected to the camera by Duo-Sync cords. Other manufacturers offer similar units. The features to look for in selecting a "dedicated" flash unit for a camera are:

1. For which camera is the unit dedicated? Independent flash unit manufacturers offer equipment suitable for specific cameras, and camera manufacturers offer flash units which will fit their own cameras.
2. Weight. The unit should be lightweight.
3. Light output. The lens apertures for TTL–OTF metering with a specific film and at a specific distance are stated in the instruction manual with the flash unit. There are some limitations. For clinical use the lens aperture number should be not less than f-8. Animals will usually be photographed at distances from 5 to 12 ft. In the close-up range where adequate depth of field is essential, apertures of f-11 at 3 ft. and f-16 at 1-1/2 to 2 ft. are desirable. The Pentax camera and flash units listed above provide these apertures with Ektachrome 200 film, the film we have selected because of its excellent color rendition of muscle and skin with electronic flash illumination. If the lens aperture numbers recommended for the flash unit under consideration are too small, there will be no recourse but to select a more powerful flash unit which may increase both the price and the weight. If the camera does not meter flash exposures through the lens, then some other type of automatic equipment is required. Many flash units have a built-in sensor which will measure the light reflected to the flash unit. These usually work well when the flash unit is mounted on the camera but are unreliable when the flash is held away from the camera. In this latter case, exposure should be controlled by a remote sensor close to the camera's optical axis and preferably clipped to the lens hood immediately above the lens. A less desirable place is the camera's flash shoe. A minor nuisance is that the sensor is connected to the flash unit by a cord. Not all flash units offer remote sensors, but if TTL–OTF metering is not used, a remote sensor should be considered to be essential, particularly in close-up photography where the flash unit is mounted to the side of the camera. At a short working distance, the field of view will be illuminated obliquely and accurate exposure can only be obtained by a sensor

mounted close to the lens. Thus, in the absence of TTL–OTF
metering, a remote sensor mounted on the camera is essential, and
a flash unit should be selected only if it has one of these.

4. Synchronizer cable connections. Dedicated flash units connected to
the camera by a Duo-Sync cord rarely disconnect or malfunction,
but the standard synchronizer cables using a so-called PC fitting to
connect the camera's shutter to the flash unit frequently do so.
These connectors press together and are held only by friction and
tend to malfunction at the most inopportune times. This problem
is well summarized by Anon (1987) who states that "PC cords are
the weakest link between flash and camera, and not much has been
done over the years to improve them. Professional photographers
. . . tend to use Paramount® replacement sync [sic] cords." These
use thicker wire and heavier terminals and plugs and are more
expensive. If PC connectors are used, they should be taped in
place. Fortunately, some camera manufacturers (e.g. Nikon) now
offer synchronizer cables that lock into the camera's body. Obviously,
the flash unit must have the same type of fitting. Use of adaptors to
connect PC cords with a new type of fitting merely perpetuates the
old problem.

5. Bracket to hold flash unit. Frequently, flash units are mounted to
the side of the camera. As we use two dedicated flash units, a
special bracket is required. The Lepp Macro-bracket system (Fig.
1.9) (Lepp & Associates, P.O. Box 6240, Los Osos, CA 93412) has
been specifically designed to allow the use of two flash units—a
main light and a fill-in light for close-up and macro-photography.
This uses either dedicated OTF flash units or manually operated
flash units. The latter have the advantage of being lightweight.
Exposure is standardized by trial for specific RR's and positions
and outputs of the two flash units. However, for larger fields (Fig.
4.58) the extension arms (Fig. 1.9) are not long enough and longer
arms would be too heavy and clumsy. In these cases the modeling
light is hand-held, either by the photographer or an assistant. The
fill-in light is mounted on the camera. The modeling light is slid
into the shoe of a standard flash bracket when the flash is not in
use. This is not only convenient and facilitates carrying the camera
and flash units but keeps the equipment from being contaminated
in the necropsy room.

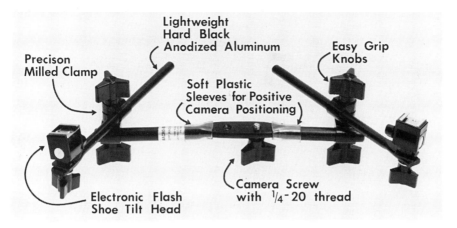

Figure 1.9. Lepp macrobracket. Courtesy of Doctor L. J. LeBeau and *Journal of Biological Photography.*

Camera

Thirty-five mm single-lens-reflex (SLR) cameras with interchangeable lenses have been used for over four decades for biological photography (Fox, 1943) and nowadays are almost universally used for specimen photography, particularly if 35mm slide transparencies are required (Vetter, 1969; Fritts, 1976). Haber (1983) "recommends the Nikon F3 as the camera of choice for pathology departments," but there is a strong element of personal preference in the selection of a SLR camera. SLR cameras have numerous advantages, but the most significant ones are accurate focusing and framing through the lens and absence of parallax error. In other words, what you see is what is recorded on film. Prior to the ready availability of convenient 35mm SLR cameras, cameras with optical viewfinders were adapted for close-up photography. These were fitted with supplementary close-up lenses and metal or wire frames known as "focal frames." The wire frames corresponded to the field of view of the lens focused at a certain distance. The correct lens-subject distance was maintained by a rod connecting the frame to the camera. Thus, the operator merely placed the frame over the area to be photographed and exposed the film, either by lights or more usually with flash. Focal frames had the advantage of simplicity and ease and quickness of use but had severe limitations. Exact focusing was not possible, and as RR's approached 1:2 where depth of field is shallow (Table IV), photographs were frequently out of focus due to small errors in positioning of the frame. Besides, the inability to check focus, shadows, specimen highlights and composition could not be evaluated. Also, if the frame was not fitted accurately and was out of position, it would appear in the picture. Even more significant was the fact that the focal frame should not be used with contaminated specimens. The frame could also damage delicate specimens. Focal frames worked well with flat surfaces such as human skin. With the advent of sophisticated and convenient SLR cameras with automatic diaphragms, focal frames became obsolete.

Features to be considered in a SLR camera are discussed below. As cameras are required for both gross anatomic specimen photography and clinical photography, desirable features for each of these will vary.

The following are desirable in a camera for gross specimen photography:

1. **Black Body**

This reduces reflections, although even black bodies will reflect in glass.

2. **Viewfinder**

1. **Eye level.** Those who use eyeglasses may prefer a high eyepoint viewfinder such as the one available for the Nikon F3 (Haber, 1983).

2. **Waist Level, With or Without a Magnifier.** Haber (1983a) uses the 6X Focusing Finder DW-4 with waist level finder of the Nikon camera. Whether an eye level or a waist level viewfinder is desirable for specimen photography will depend on the height of the camera on a vertical stand in relation to the operator's eye. With our equipment we use only the eye level finder and a step stool to allow the operator to see through the viewfinder, when the camera is elevated (Fig. 1.4). However, for a camera mounted on a copy stand on a bench and used to photograph laboratory animals or small specimens, the waist level finder may be more convenient.

3. **Focusing Screen.** This should be similar to the Nikon E screen which is a ground glass screen with horizontal and vertical lines to aid in orienting specimens. Focusing can take place on any part of the screen (Fig. 1.10).

Factors to consider in the selection of a viewfinder are brightness of the image, curvature of the borders which makes framing difficult, and accuracy of the area visible in the viewfinder compared to the area recorded on film. Viewfinders vary considerably in brightness between different cameras even with lenses of the same aperture. As most macro-

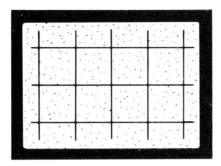

Figure 1.10. Nikon E focusing screen. Focusing can be done anywhere on the screen, a real advantage in close-up photography. The grid lines aid in alignment of specimens such as brain slices.

lenses have relatively small maximum apertures (e.g. f-2.8 or f-3.5), a bright viewfinder is an advantage, as it facilitates focusing. In some models the edge of the viewfinder appears curved and makes it very difficult to place the ruler squarely along the lower edge.

A significant factor is viewfinder accuracy (i.e. the relationship between the size of the image seen in the viewfinder compared to the actual size of the image on film). Some viewfinders are highly accurate, others make allowance for the 2mm to 3mm of 2 × 2 transparencies covered by the mask, but some cheaper cameras are quite inaccurate and include more image on the film than is visible in the viewfinder. Reasonably high accuracy is required for the framing of gross specimens. If transparencies are to be used for television, focusing screens with grids to indicate the margins of the television screens as well as for film strip and 4 × 5 films are available (Photographic-Lee, 909 Micheltorena Street, Los Angeles, California 90026).

Another factor that affects ease of focusing is the magnification of the viewfinder. Formerly, these all had a 1X or 0.95X magnification, but as manufacturers have included more and more data on shutter speed, aperture, exposure compensation, etc., in automated and semi-automated cameras, they have reduced the magnification of the focusing screen to allow the eye to see both screen and data displays easily. Magnification factors of the viewfinders of different models of Pentax cameras vary between 0.67X and 0.95X. Reduction in magnification makes focusing more difficult, particularly under marginal conditions such as occur in dim light. Thus, the prospective purchaser would be wise to check the ease of focusing under the proposed conditions of use.

3. Shutter

Most modern single lens reflex cameras have an adequate range of speeds, particularly slow speeds up to half or one second. This is a desirable feature, as slow shutter speeds may be necessary to give the correct exposure with small apertures such as f-16, required to obtain adequate depth of field with RR's used in close-up photography. There are still some cameras whose shutter-speed dial rotates during exposure. If this is restrained accidently by hand or a strap during exposure, shutter speeds will be inaccurate. Shutter dials should not be easily dislodged accidentally from one speed setting to another. This is essential in our technique where the shutter speed is kept constant. Cameras with focal plane shutters synchronize with electronic flash only when both shutter curtains are completely open. The shutter speed at which this occurs varies with different cameras and has been progressively increased from 1/30 second to 1/125 second or faster over the last couple of decades. A fast shutter synchronization speed is desirable, as it reduces the chances of ambient lighting recording on the film, as for example from the overhead lights in the necropsy room. Thus, desirable features are a range of shutter speeds from 1/1000 to 1/2 or 1 second, a non-rotating shutter dial which is not easily dislodged accidentally, and synchronization with electronic flash at 1/125 second or faster.

4. Automatic Exposure

Although a high degree of exposure automation is now available in cameras, it is less successful with many gross specimens than with conventional subjects. Calibration of meters in cameras is based on the assumption that a conventional subject reflects 18 percent of the light that falls on it. This is certainly not true of such subjects as bleached fixed brain slices supported over a black background or a black animal against a light grey wall. The ratio of the areas occupied by the white specimen and the black background markedly influences the exposure determined by automatic equipment. Therefore, for photography of gross specimens, we use a camera without automatic exposure and determine exposure by standardization of the lamps.

5. Lens

When macro-lenses were first introduced, cameras were selected based on the availability of this type of lens. However, nowadays highly corrected "macro" or "micro" lenses, as they are sometimes called, are available for a wide variety of SLR cameras. In contrast to conventional lenses, these lenses are highly corrected for the close-up range rather than when focused at infinity, and they have focusing mounts that allow extension of the lens so that the maximum size of the image on the film plane can be as much a half of that of the real subject. This ratio between the length of the subject and the length of its image on film is called the ratio of reproduction (RR) and in the case described equals 1:2. Many macro-lenses have a removable extension tube (sometimes called a "repro" tube) to allow focusing of life-sized images, RR = 1:1. Unfortunately, many macro-lenses have relatively small maximum apertures; f-2.8 or f-3.5 are common, which reduces the brightness of the image in the viewfinder. However, this is rarely a difficulty in specimen photography.

Macro-lenses are available in different focal lengths from 50mm to 55mm (normal) up to 90mm to 105mm. The latter have a smaller angle of acceptance than "normal" lenses, and therefore to include the same field (same RR) as a 50mm lens, the free working (lens-subject) distance has to be increased. This has the advantage of giving "better" (i.e. less distorted) perspective at extreme close-ups and increasing the working distance and thus the safety margin when photographing infectious or obnoxious material or unpredictable live animals. Haber (1983b) states that the 50mm f-2.8 Micro-Nikkor, 105mm f-4 Micro-Nikkor, and the 200mm f-4 Micro-Nikkor for the Nikon camera are excellent. He considers the 55mm f-2.8 Micro-Nikkor to be "one of the sharpest lenses made" (Haber, 1982). Nikon's Medical-Nikkor 120mm f-4 IF lens is capable of photographing from RR's of 1:11 to 1:1 and has a built-in focusing lamp and a ring flash for cavity photography. The 50mm macro-lens is the most versatile choice for a camera mounted on a vertical-mounted camera stand, as it can cover both large and small specimens.

At RR's of approximately 1:4 and less, the working distance becomes so small that there can be distortion. In these cases, a longer focal length macro-lens (e.g. 105mm) would give better results. Besides macro-lenses of a single focal length, there are also macro-zoom lenses. These have the advantage that at a fixed working distance, the size of the image (RR) can be varied by changing the focal length (zooming). This is a desirable feature when the viewpoint cannot be moved, as for example during surgery or in cadaver photography. Haber (1983) has pointed out that compared with macro-lenses, macro-zoom lenses have the following disadvantages:

1. larger and heavier.
2. maximum aperture is smaller. This is only important if it is necessary to focus in dim light.

3. very often the largest magnification is a reproduction ratio (RR) of 1:4. Most single focal length macro-lenses can reach RR = 1:2 or even RR = 1:1.
4. generally more expensive.
5. less sharp, usually in the corners, although this may not be detectable at f-11.

For specimen photography with a vertically mounted camera on a photographic stand, Haber (1983) is convinced that the disadvantages listed above are more important than the minor convenience of being able to change the image size (RR) by zooming, particularly when moving the camera up or down on a vertical stand is so easy. However, the macro-zoom lens is useful in cadaver and clinical photography.

6. Automatically Compensating Diaphragms

An annoying feature of close-up photography is that the marked apertures on the lens (e.g. f-8, f-11) are no longer optically true and do not transmit the same amount of light once the RR is less than approximately 1:10 (Table IX). This corresponds to a field size of 15 × 10 inches for a 35mm camera whose frame is 1-½ × 1 inches. Thus, in close-up photographs, the amount of light transmitted to the film plane at a specific aperture (e.g. f-16) is reduced at RR's less than 1:10 than when the lens is focused on infinity with a subject of constant reflectance. Exposure correction factors, called "close-up factors" or "bellows factors," are necessary to adjust for this discrepancy and become increasingly larger, and thus more important, as the RR approaches one. Automatic exposure cameras with through-the-lens (TTL) metering automatically compensate for this defect.

However, in the absence of this type of metering, correction has to be done manually. Exposure correction tables are available. Some macro-lenses have distance, RR and exposure correction factors marked on the lens focusing mount. However, in the mid 1960s, Nikon introduced an f-3.5 Micro-Nikkor lens (lens numbers from 220,000 to 273,000) which had an automatically compensating diaphragm (Fig. 1.11). This was described in the instruction booklet (Nippon Kogaku, 1969) "as another distinctive feature the lens is provided, in addition to the automatic pre-set aperture diaphragm, with an automatic aperture compensating device which provides an image of constant brightness regardless of . . . magnification thus requiring . . . no exposure factors in close-up photography." As this remarkable lens was focused from infinity to RR = 1:2, the lens aperture automatically increased in diameter so that the amount of light transmitted at a marked aperture was constant. Thus, the lens passed the same amount of light at f-16, whether the lens was focused at infinity or RR = 1:2, from a subject with constant reflectance. Such a feature is not an advantage with cameras that meter exposure through the lens (TTL) and the automatically compensating diaphragm was discontinued. For cameras used with standardized light sources (as in copy work), the automatically compensating diaphragm completely eliminated the need for exposure correction at different ratios of reproduction —an enormous advantage which has been favorably commented on by Vetter (1969). We have had a recent model of the 55mm f-2.8 Micro-Nikkor lens custom-fitted with an automatically compensating diaphragm by Professional Camera Repair Service (37 West 47th Street, New York, NY 10036). The modification is relatively inexpensive but is an enormous advantage with standardized lighting.

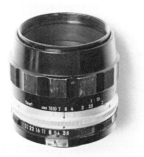

Figure 1.11. A 55mm f-3.5 Micro-Nikkor lens with automatically compensating diaphragm which is invaluable in facilitating copy work and close-up photography with fixed lighting and standardized exposures.

Other features to look for in a lens include:

1. smallest aperture, f-22 is usually adequate, but f-32 can be useful occasionally.
2. "click" stops with clicks or detents at all half-stop intervals. To obtain adequate depth of field, macro-lenses are frequently used at apertures between f-11 and f-22. Half stops are essential for fine-tuning exposures, particularly of white subjects such as bones and fixed brain slices where there is little exposure latitude. Some macro-lenses do not have click stops between full stops and some do not have them between f-11, 16, and 22. In the absence of click

stops, setting the aperture between full stops can be unreliable, as the aperture may be moved when the automatic diaphragm closes during exposure. Loomis (1984) described a procedure for adding "click" half stops to 55mm and 105mm Micro-Nikkor lenses.

3. ease of focusing which depends on how far the lens barrel has to be rotated.

4. ease of removal and insertion of interchangeable lenses.

7. Cable Release

This relatively inexpensive item can be a nuisance. It needs to be black to prevent reflections and long enough so that the photographer's hand is not reflected in the specimen glass and vibrations are not transmitted to the camera. However, if it is too long, the end may touch specimens as the camera focuses close to RR = 1:1, thus becoming contaminated. A locking cable release is not only not required but also has the disadvantage of locking unexpectedly, keeping the exposure release depressed. Thus, a cable release should be selected for flexibility and adequate length (approximately 8 inches), but it should not touch specimens when the camera is focused to RR = 1:2.

Desirable features in a camera for clinical photography are similar to those discussed above with the following differences.

1. Automatic Exposure Control

For clinical photography using available light, it is helpful to have this option. It speeds photography, particularly when lighting levels fluctuate as can occur outdoors on a partially overcast day. Most advanced SLR cameras offer several types of automatic exposure control, e.g. programmed, aperture priority and shutter priority.

2. Lens

For clinical work, the working (lens-subject) distance of a lens is of critical importance. In photography of small animals such as dogs to be able to fill the frame but to stay back several feet from the subject requires a long focal length lens. A 105mm lens is excellent for small animal photography. A zoom lens with a 35mm to 135mm range offers more flexibility and allows the photographer to fill the frame with different-sized animals at different working distances.

3. Dedicated TTL-OTF Flash Exposure Control

This feature was described above under "Flash Equipment" and is essential to allow the use of twin flashes with accurate automatic exposure control.

Film

The choice of a color film always involves a considerable subjective component and personal preference. Hurtgen (1978) has listed factors to be considered in the selection of a color film for medical photography. These include (1) color balance, (2) film speed (sensitivity, ISO rating), (3) reciprocity characteristics, (4) format, (5) processing, (6) resolving power, (7) granularity value and (8) personal preference and convenience. Another category that could be added is (9) stability of dyes during storage or exposure to light.

Color Balance. This is the name given to the type of light source to which the color film has been matched or balanced. There are 3 major types: type A film balanced for 3400°K light (photoflood lamps), type B film for 3200°K (studio lamps), and daylight film balance for 5500°K light—the approximate color temperature of noonday light and electronic flash.

Film Speed. The photographic jargon for a film's sensitivity to light is "speed." It is expressed by an ISO (formally ASA) number or rating and is arithmetic. In other words, a 100 ISO film is twice as "fast" or sensitive as a 50 ISO film. The film speed is often intimately associated with other film characteristics such as resolving power and granularity value and thus a slow film such as Kodachrome 40 may be selected because of its desirable high resolution and low granularity. However, if fast exposures are required to "freeze" subject motion or allow adequate depth of field, or both, then a fast film with a higher ISO rating will have to be selected, even if this means some lack of quality due to poorer resolution and higher granularity. For inanimate subjects in a studio, subject or camera motion is not a factor and thus the film should be selected to obtain the highest quality image. This generally means a slow film, unless the lighting is inadequate which would result in exposures which would be so long as to produce reciprocity failure.

Reciprocity Failure. The reciprocity law states that: $E = IT$ where $E =$ total exposure, $I =$ illumination, $T =$ time. Thus E, the total amount of light energy, could be delivered to the film either by a low-intensity light (I) for a long period (T), or a high-intensity light (I) for a short period (T) (Fig. 1.12). The law holds true for a wide range of shutter speeds and manufacturers publish those speeds at which their films start to develop reciprocity failure. It is an important consideration in color films, as in these, reciprocity failure is expressed as color casts as well as underexposure. Most films do not show reciprocity failure between 1/1000 second and 1/10 second, and thus a shutter speed within this range should be chosen to avoid color casts from reciprocity failure.

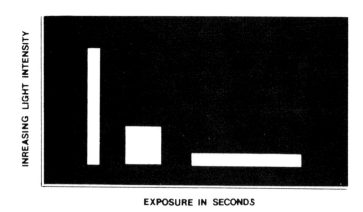

Figure 1.12. The amount of light reaching the film is the same in the above three cases: a very intense light for a brief exposure time (*left*), a moderately intense light for a medium exposure time (*middle*) and a dim light for a long exposure (*right*). The response of the film is not always the same, as very brief and very long exposures cause reciprocity failure.

Format. Hurtgen (1978) has summarized the situation by stating that "if slides are required for projection, a transparency film such as Kodachrome should be used." If color prints are desired, a color negative film is the logical choice, because although color slides can be made from color negative film and prints can be made from color transparencies, for each conversion there is a small loss of quality. Thus, if the principal purpose is to obtain a slide for projection, then color transparency film should be used.

Processing. Some films such as Ektachrome can be processed by the user or local laboratories and can be ready in hours. However, Kodachrome must be shipped to a processing laboratory, a procedure that may take days or even longer.

Resolving Power and Granularity Value. Resolving power is the ability of a film or lens to separate adjacent pairs of lines, and the results are expressed as lines/mm, with test-object contrasts of 1000:1 and 1.6:1 representing high and low contrast subjects, respectively (Hurtgen, 1978). The resolving power of Kodak films is listed in Table VI. The resolving power of good quality camera lenses is over 100 lines/mm, even though the theoretical resolving power may be much higher (Table V). Thus, the film rather than the lens is frequently the limiting factor in resolution.

Graininess is the appearance of non-uniform densities in what should be a uniformly dense area such as the sky or skin tones. It is related to the size of the silver grains in the emulsion. Fast films have larger grains and tend to be grainier than slow films. Hence, slow films should be selected whenever possible for the photography of specimens.

Personal Preference Including Color Rendition. Factors include convenience and speed of processing, cost of film (particularly if this is available in bulk), availability, and, most important, the perception of the rendition of colors, particularly those of skin and tissue. For example, using flash illumination, Ektachrome 200 renders flesh tones and muscle with remarkable fidelity. Therefore, when the color of flesh tones is a principal requirement, this film should be selected, even though its resolving power and granularity value are inferior to those of a slow speed film such as Kodachrome 25.

Stability of the Dyes Under Storage and Exposure to Light. These data are published by film manufacturers. One film may be very resistant to fading when projected repeatedly, while another may have little color shift in dyes after decades of storage under optimal conditions. Thus, the former film should be selected for slide shows with continued projection over weeks or months and the second film for archival storage.

We prefer Kodachrome 40 for color photography of gross specimens because of its color fidelity, resolution, low graininess and stability of the dyes on storage. Vetter (1984) uses Ektachrome EPY, a 50 ISO tungsten film. For clinical and necropsy specimens photographed with electronic flash, we use Ektachrome 200 because of its realistic rendition of flesh colors. Haber (1984) prefers Kodachrome 64, but our electronic flash produces a bluish cast with this film. Film speed is often a major consideration in the selection of a film. If the intensity of illumination from the lamps is inadequate, exposures with slow films may be so long as to cause reciprocity failure and thus color casts. In the designing of facilities it is critical that films should not be chosen to suit lamps, but photographic lamps should be chosen because they have sufficient intensity and correct color temperature to allow the optimum film to be used at an aperture which is the best compromise between resolution and depth of field, and at a shutter speed at which there is no reciprocity failure. Thus, selection of the correct lamp directly influences the film that can be used.

Monochrome Photography of Gross Specimens. Slow films are required because as with slow color films, they have high resolution, low granularity indices and excellent acutance. Acutance is an index of the sharpness of lines between light and dark areas, and high acutance increases the appearance of sharpness. Slow black-and-white films are characteristically very contrasty, although Kodak Panatomic X (ISO 32) is an exception and is of medium contrast. Efke (Adox) KB-14 has slightly more contrast than Panatomic X. In the same way that fast color films may be required to "freeze" subject motion, so will fast black-and-white films be required for these subjects. Marshall and Marshall (1975) used Ilford Pan F 35mm film. They state that any difference in quality in prints up to 8 × 6 inches in size, whether from large format or 35mm negatives, should be undetectable. For cadaver photography with available room light, a film with a long tonal gradation such as Kodak Tri-X (ISO 400) should be selected, because the tonal gradation is more important than the lower resolving power and increased graininess. These latter features may not be evident in small prints used for publication.

Thus, the selection of a film is a compromise among the above factors. In planning facilities, it is essential that lamps be selected with sufficiently intense illumination to allow the use of slow films which are most likely to produce the highest quality images.

Dissection Equipment and Supplies

The presence of retractors or clamps in photographs is distracting and should be avoided if possible. Occasionally, there is no alternative, but fortunately nowadays surgical suppliers have developed instruments with a special low-glare finish for use with television. These have a less reflective surface than conventional stainless steel instruments and are less distracting in photographs. Instruments that may be included in photographs include Allis clamps, Gelpi retractors and urinary catheters. Other instruments that should be kept on hand for dissection and preparation of specimens in the photography room include 8 inch straight Mayo scissors, 6 inch plain and 6 inch rat-tooth tissue forceps, scalpel handles with #22 and #60 scalpel blades, funnels of different sizes for intratracheal perfusion, bowel clamps to clamp tracheas of small animals and sutures and needles.

Knives. Long-bladed knives are essential to be able to slice organs with one motion and so avoid serrations on the cut surface. Useful knives include:

- R. H. Forschner Co., Switzerland, Catalog No. 109-14, knife, 14 inches long, slightly curved
- Lipshaw Manufacturing Co., Detroit, Michigan 48210, Catalog No. 715, postmortem knife, 18 × 1 × ⅛ inches.
- Feather Industries Limited, Tokyo, Japan, Labtron Scientific Corporation, 91 Cabot Court, Hauppauge, NY. 11788, Catalog No. 325, disposable brain knife blade, 450mm (18 inches) with Catalog No. 00535 plastic handle (Fig. 4.20).
- Thomas Scientific, P. O. Box 779, Philadelphia, PA 19105-0779, Catalog No. 6727-C20, Blade, tissue slicer, 4-⅝ × ¾ inches, disposable.

Gloves. As has been discussed under "Specimen Preparation," occasionally the only reasonable way to orient and retract the sides of a specimen (e.g. heart to reveal a lesion) is by holding it between gloved hands. Gloves should always be worn, both because of the possibility of infection and also because the texture of human skin and the excellence or otherwise of the manicure distracts attention from the main subject. The least distracting gloves are natural latex. Colored gloves such as red, green, blue, yellow and black should not be used. Semitransparent gloves reveal the wearer's skin texture and hair. The presence of rings and wristwatches on the prosector, besides indicating poor technique, is distracting. Grey, disposable polyethylene gloves are too pale and thus distracting. Gloves should fit well so that unsightly folds and creases do not form. Consequently, different-sized gloves must be available in the photography room.

Retractors. To expose the lumens of relatively rigid viscera such as the heart, larynx or trachea, some form of retraction is required. To do this neatly without distractive props is not easy. Methods that have been used include:

1. pinning the specimen with thumbtacks (drawing pins), plastic-headed stick pins, sewing pins or even hypodermic needles to a cork or wooden background.
2. sutures placed in the edges of the specimen attached to glass rods or to pins outside the field of view.

3. some makeshift type of spreader such as wooden applicator sticks (orange sticks), tongue depressors, 1 × 3 inch glass microscope slides and even hypodermic needles.
4. surgical retractors such as a Gelpi retractor.
5. hand-held.

Usually pinning is undesirable, as the pins damage the edge of the specimen with rows of holes (Martin, 1961) and sutures through the edge stretch the wall unnaturally at the point of attachment. Makeshift props such as those listed above are distracting. Stainless steel surgical retractors are also distracting because of their gleaming surfaces, and usually the jaws or handles extend beyond the frame and lead the eye out of the picture. Low-glare stainless steel instruments designed for television are better. Although stainless steel retractors are somewhat distracting, they have the advantages of being neat, easy to use, and more aesthetically pleasing than many of the makeshift retractors.

Retracting walls of specimens and maintaining their correct orientation can be done easily by hands when it is impossible for mechanical retractors. This is particularly true of the chambers of the heart. Thus, some photographers use gloved hands to do this. The image of the hands can be opaqued out of the negative, but hands covered by well-fitting surgical gloves are far more acceptable in a photograph than strings running out of the field of view or makeshift props. Gloved hands are readily accepted in color transparencies, but the amount visible should be kept to a minimum. Obviously, the gloves should not be distracting and must be scrupulously clean, well fitting, have no printing visible, be a natural latex color and not be too transparent, as this reveals the caliber of the manicure. Kennedy (1987) designed a traction frame of clear Plexiglas® used to pull open rigid fixed organs such as heart and intestine. The frame is made in the same proportions as the camera's frame (1:1.5 in the case of 35mm camera). Sutures of black 00 or 000 silk are sewn through the back of the specimens and the sutures passed to the edge of the frame where they are attached by sliding them under cleats. Used with a black background, the sutures are virtually invisible. In monochrome photography with large negatives, pins and threads can be opaqued out, but it is usually impossible to do this for internally placed retractors.

Another completely different approach is to try to dissect the specimen so that retractors are unnecessary. These attempts are not always successful, and thus sequential photographs are needed so that if the later attempts are unsatisfactory, earlier photographs are available. One method of exposing the luminal surface of a rigid tube such as the trachea is to dissect off the upper half and expose the lower half. This technique results in approximately the same area of specimen being visible to the camera and, at the same time, no retractors are required. The procedure is less acceptable when it destroys landmarks. Then a Gelpi retractor is more suitable. The larynx can be spread apart by a Gelpi retractor or alternatively by sutures through the outer walls. The photograph should be framed to show only the interior of the larynx.

If natural latex covered metal retractors were available, they would be the simplest and least distracting method for exposing the lumens of many organs. However, orientation of some organs such as the heart to show valves and chambers is so complicated, particularly in a hypertrophic heart after fixation, that retraction by gloved hands is the simplest and easiest way to obtain good results.

Props. Frequently, specimens will need to be propped into position, for example, to raise the surface of a kidney parallel to the film plane. Most of the adjustments will be small, and a compressible material such as modeling clay (plasticine) functions very well. It can also be used to elevate rulers. An unobtrusive color such as dark grey is preferred in case some accidentally becomes visible to the camera. Modeling clay tends to cling and leave fine remnants, and thus rulers should always be cleaned carefully. The problem with remnants does not occur so readily with some of the modern caulking compounds such as Mortite® (Editors, 1987) (Mortell Co., Kankakee, IL 60901). Weather stripping and caulking cord is available in dark brown. Both modeling clay and Mortite leave dull marks on glass backgrounds after removal.

Miscellaneous Items. These include:

- grey modeling clay or Mortite weather stripping (Mortell Co., Kankakee, IL 60901)
- wooden blocks painted flat black, measuring $3 \times 2 \times 1/2$ inches, $3 \times 2 \times 3/4$ inches, $3 \times 2 \times 1$ inches and $3 \times 2 \times 2$ inches
- $1/8$ inch thick lead blocks, painted flat black
- glass cleaner
- laboratory towels, soft, low-lint, disposable (Kaydry EX–L®)
- physiological saline
- Jores' solution
- neutral buffered 10% formalin (10% NBF)
- immersion tank and large Petri dishes (see "Specular Highlights")

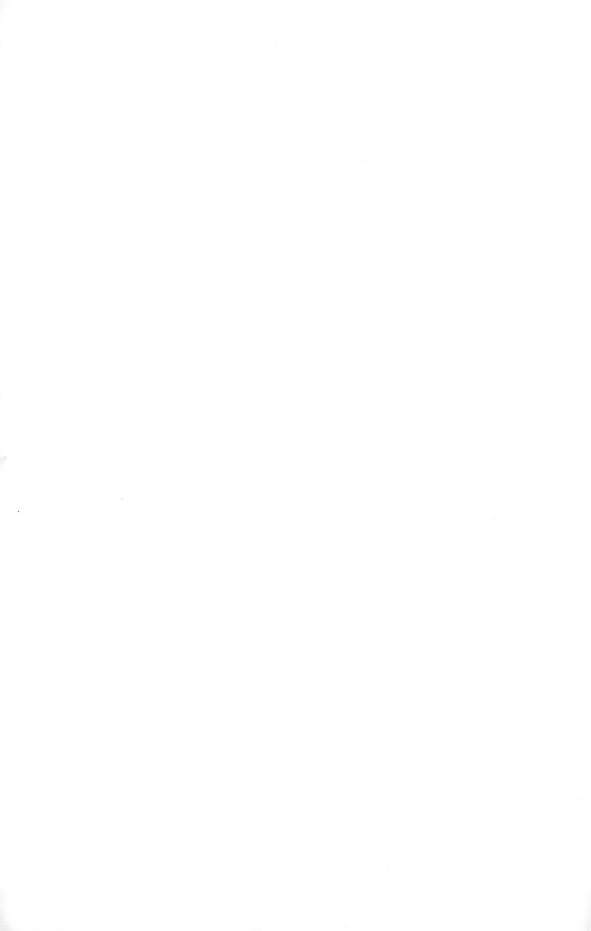

Chapter 2

BACKGROUNDS AND ACCESSORIES

In portraiture, the problem of shadows cast on the background is overcome by first lighting the subject to obtain the desired effect, placing the background sufficiently far away to be out of sharp focus and then lighting it independently. To do this, there must be sufficient space between subject and background to allow shadows to fall outside the field of view of the camera, or to be illuminated by separate lights. This same technique should apply to photography of pathological specimens, but, because the camera is mounted vertically, space between the specimen and background is limited. Large specimens require larger backgrounds and thus longer working distances which may result in the camera being inconveniently high. Various compromises have been made. Optimal lighting of specimens has been altered to control the placement of background shadows (Marshall, 1957). Backgrounds have been selected to minimize shadows rather than to present the specimen optimally. This is exemplified by the use of black backgrounds for transparencies and white backgrounds for monochrome photographs of all specimens, despite the fact that the occasions when absolutely black or blank white backgrounds are really complementary to the subject are rare.

Earliest anatomic drawings were embellished with backgrounds of landscapes or ornamental scenes (Marshal, 1957). Such ancillary detail may be of historical interest now centuries later but does not enhance the appearance of the specimen. Today, a homogeneous background, with no detail except a scale, is desired. The major difficulties are controlling cast shadows and selecting the grey scale (tonal) value of the background to suit the subject. Because of the distracting effect of unsuitable backgrounds, an extensive literature has developed. There have been discussions on the desirability of colored versus uncolored, white versus black and various tones of grey and opaque versus transparent. Despite all the discussions which will be reviewed below, the fact remains that even today, backgrounds in many photographs are still unsuitable and a

43

convenient shadowless background whose tone can be varied from white through greys to black is still not available for large pathological specimens.

The criteria for judging backgrounds have been succinctly described by Halsman (1955) who stated that "background must always be subservient to the subject in hue (name of color), brightness (grey scale value) and saturation (purity of color) and thus must not compete for attention or falsely affect the interpretation of the specimens." Blaker (1977a) declared that the purposes of a background are to:

1. isolate the subject.
2. avoid distraction and clutter.
3. be impossible to confuse with the subject.
4. be suitable for printing in publications.

Backgrounds according to Martinsen (1952) fall into three classes, depending on the subjects to be photographed:

1. live subjects (portraits)
2. dead subjects (cadavers)
3. gross pathological specimens

Backgrounds for pathological specimens will be discussed here. Backgrounds for live subjects and cadavers are described later. The basic types of backgrounds are white, grey, black, colored, and natural. All of these have limitations and advantages. A black background has the advantage of producing a strong tonal contrast between subject and background and emphasizing outline (Gibson, 1950), but a black background may be at a serious disadvantage on the printed page, where it may reproduce as a grey rather than a black in all but the highest quality printing. Choice of a background is strongly influenced by whether the photograph is to be a color transparency for projection in a darkened room or a monochrome print for a publication. A white or very light grey background is often very suitable for black-and-white prints, but a white background is glaring and extremely distracting in projected transparencies.

WHITE BACKGROUNDS

These have the advantage in monochrome prints of:

• reproducing best in publications
• isolating the subject
• are practical and easy to obtain (Blaker, 1977a)

White backgrounds reproduce as faint grey on the printed page (Blaker, 1977a). For a background to record as white in a print, it has to receive illumination in addition to that falling on the specimen. The usual recommendation is to have twice the light (incident light) falling on the white background than on the subject, unless the subject is very dark (Blaker, 1977a). Kodak (1970) recommends that the light *reflected* from the background should be three times that *reflected* from the specimen. The white background will record on the shoulder of the characteristic (d log E) curve of the negative, while the subject is on the straight line portion. However, there are precautions to be taken. Those portions of the white background not included in the photograph should be masked off to prevent flare (Blaker, 1977a), which is non-image forming light that degrades the contrast of the image in the camera. This is a real danger and is most likely to occur if the background is too large or too bright. As a guide, flare is likely to develop if the background area is greater than the subject area or is twice as bright (Blaker, 1977a). Another problem with excessively light backgrounds is light reflecting from the contours of the subject, for example, the sides of the fingers of a human hand can be over-illuminated (Haberlein, 1979). Therefore, light boxes should have masks to limit the extent of the lighted background and dimmers to control the intensity of the background illumination.

Techniques to Obtain White Backgrounds (Blaker, 1965a)

1. The simplest method is to use a light box of the transmitted light variety. Separate lights are used to illuminate the specimen. The ratio of the background to specimen illumination should be adjusted, usually to 3:1. The light reflected from the specimen from the top lights should be measured with the light box turned off, but the light from the light box should be metered with both the top and light box lights on.
2. Heavy-duty aluminum foil, matte side up, placed immediately under the specimen can be used if there is axial lighting. This method is inapplicable to photography of most specimens.
3. Skylight from an overcast sky. Such lighting results in a diffuse low contrast lighting and requires that the negative receive additional development to increase contrast. This results in a white background recording as white or extremely light grey in the print. Usually, the specimen is supported on a glass above a white card.

Obviously, such an arrangement is makeshift and is dependent on the availability and vagaries of skylight.

BLACK BACKGROUNDS

As Blaker (1977a) states, "for sheer drama of presentation, ... black backgrounds are unbeatable in either color or black and white." The winning color transparencies in competitions of gross specimens frequently have black backgrounds (American Society of Clinical Pathologists, 1982). Black backgrounds have the following advantages:

- maximum impact
- easy to obtain, either with black velvet or a black box
- no problem with shadows or unevenly illuminated backgrounds
- color casts are obscured
- emphasis is on the outline of the subject, particularly if this is light colored or light toned

Black backgrounds have maximum impact in projected images; the subject seems to "float" in a black void, but there are significant disadvantages. Black is a funereal "color," psychologically depressing and, when used exclusively, "provides a mood of boredom and gloom" (Haeberlein, 1979). Viewing a continuous stream of transparencies with black backgrounds with high contrast, high impact and accentuation of the outline is not only fatiguing (Harris, 1956) but the viewer's eye is constantly attracted back to the junction of the specimen and background. Thus, the rest of the specimen and important internal detail may be ignored by the viewer. Halsman (1955) has summed up the problem by saying that "high contrast will make the specimen as a whole stand out from the background, but it will result in 'harder seeing' of fine detail within the specimen." Also, black backgrounds are less suitable for very dark specimens because the borders tend to merge with the background. In prints, they are of limited use (Blaker, 1977a), because black only reproduces well in high-quality printing and defects such as patches of uneven tone, breaks and spots are easily visible. Also, in the same way that the border of the specimen and background is emphasized, so is the junction of the black print and the surrounding white paper. This distracts attention from the subject. Psychologically, the prints can be depressing because they recall black-edged bereavement notices.

Techniques for Obtaining Black Backgrounds

Black backgrounds are obtained by using two basic methods:

1. **An Almost Totally Non-reflective Background.** Deep-nap velvet is recommended. Such backgrounds are expensive and easily contaminated by animal hair, dandruff, etc. and are generally unsuitable for wet or infectious specimens. Cho (1983, Pers. Com.) has used black velvet remnants as disposable backgrounds for gross specimens. LeBeau and Wimmer (1982) recommend black glass highly if the incident light is at a low angle to prevent light being reflected from the glass into the lens. Black glass is made by spraying one side of a glass sheet with flat black paint. The specimen is placed on the other side. The results are excellent and the background is almost totally black.

2. **Glass Topped "Black Box"** (Fig. 2.1). The principle is simple; the inside of the box is so deep that no light falls on the bottom and it is painted black or lined with black velvet (Blaker, 1977a; Vetter, 1969). The box works well for gross specimens. With a 50mm lens on a 35mm camera (45° acceptance angle), the edges of the box are illuminated by lights and may be included in the photograph and thus these sides must be matte black. Alternatively, a longer focal length lens (e.g. 90mm with an acceptance angle of 22.5°) could be used as it views less of the walls (Fig. 2.2).

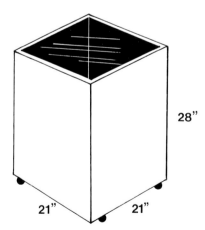

28"

21"   21"

Figure 2.1. Black box. This is made of wood, painted flat black on the inside and has a glass top which is easily lifted out for cleaning.

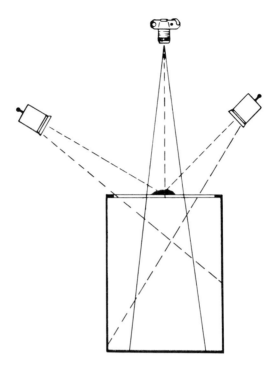

Figure 2.2. Black box. With small specimens, the camera views only the bottom of the box which is not illuminated by the photographic lamps, ensuring a black background.

An obvious tendency is to make the box large enough to accommodate all specimens, but there are physical limits. Large boxes will not leave much space to move the box to left or right between the lights or towards or away from the wall to allow centering of the specimen. After considerable experimentation we have found that a box whose outside dimensions are 22 × 22 inches with an overall height, including castors (from floor to glass), of 28 inches and with a top glass of 21 × 21 inches is suitable for most of our specimens with the standardized lighting arrangement. The optimal height of the box, and thus the specimen supported on its surface, depends on the working height of the camera and this is obviously dependent on the size of the specimen. The camera is positioned lower for small and higher for large specimens. The camera position is also controlled by the focal length of the lens, and at RR = 1:1 a 50mm lens has a working (lens-subject) distance of 4 inches. With a 28 inch high box, the camera's viewfinder is approximately 33 inches from the floor, which is quite convenient.

Specifications. The box illustrated in Figure 2.1, has the following features:

- glass $21 \times 21 \times \frac{1}{4}$ inches with smooth edges to protect fingers
- rigid, $\frac{5}{8}$ inch plywood walls and base
- two semicircular finger holes cut at each end to facilitate lifting out of the glass
- overall height including castors 28 inches
- castors need to be adjustable if floor is not level
- painted flat black inside
- painted light grey glossy washable on the outside
- a wooden ledge of $\frac{1}{4} \times \frac{1}{2}$ inches wood is attached $\frac{3}{16}$ inches from the top. This is to support the glass whose top surface should be slightly above the level of the side of the box to facilitate cleaning.

This box has worked very well. The glass is easily removed for cleaning and is sufficiently large, so that if small specimens ooze they can be moved to another area for photography. Maintenance of the box is minimal. The inside has to be sprayed with flat black paint occasionally and the glass cleaned regularly and replaced when scratched. Cleaning of the glass is described below.

For the cadavers of laboratory animals and small specimens, the box designed by Vetter (1969) to fit on a laboratory bench may be more suitable. This measures $17 \times 21 \times 6$ inches and is lined with black velvet. The black background is due to the non-reflectivity of the velvet rather than the depth of the box. We recommend a square box which does not unconsciously bias the photographer to place long specimens in the horizontal format to fit the shape of the box, rather than in their correct anatomic position.

The major advantage of the black box background is that it is extremely easy to use. Cast shadows are absent and the whole of the top glass plate is available to hold the specimen, because the black walls of the box also act as a background. This is in contrast to light boxes where the background itself is some distance below the specimen and thus the useful area of the top glass is reduced. Smears of dried exudates on glass are not as obvious with black backgrounds as they are with transilluminated light ones. Even if a full black is not produced on the transparency, a very dark grey background is excellent and may be superior, because contrast between the specimen and the background is reduced. Such dark grey backgrounds may be produced by shallow boxes lined by black velvet or by black cloth. Thus, the black background is the easiest to use.

It produces dramatic pictures with impact, has considerable audience acceptance and consequently is popular with photographers. However, its use is best reserved for those specimens in which it is necessary to show dramatic changes in outline, and unfortunately such specimens are a minority.

COLORED BACKGROUNDS

One of the major debates over the last 30 years has been on the desirability or undesirability of colored backgrounds, particularly in gross specimen photography. Advantages cited include (Kodak, 1966):

1. Visibility of important black, white or grey areas which would be lost against a black, white or grey background, respectively.
2. Vividness and clarity of the subject.

However, the major criticism has been that colored backgrounds falsify the viewer's perception of the specimen and, as Halsman (1955) has pointed out: "If (the perceptions of) colors are visually strengthened by the use of complementary backgrounds, then the (perceptions of) colors within the specimen are falsified." Jenny et al. (1981) evaluated and illustrated the effect of yellow, blue and red backgrounds on the perception of yellowish ammonite and found that "strong color contrasts may seem attractive at first, but the complementary colors may lead to appreciable falsification of the colors of the object. . . . The complementary color blue exaggerates the yellow tone. . . . For scientific documentation purposes, the best background colors are white, grey or black." Other examples of this type of change are presented by Kodak (1966). For the most critical work (for example, comparing color plates), a totally neutral background is recommended by the Committee on Colorimetry, Optical Society of America (Halsman, 1955). Those advocating colored backgrounds usually recommend a color complementary to the major color of the specimen. As most tissues are pinkish, a bluish-green is frequently chosen (Kodak, 1966), although Beiter and Bohrod (1944) recommend "some shade of blue." For the same reason, bluish-green has been recommended as a background for photographs of caucasian skin (Gibson, 1950). There is no good reason for its use in clinical photographs in veterinary medicine, as animals vary widely in coat color. The combination of a bluish-green background with black, dark brown or dark red hair is not a happy choice. There is even less justification for the use of yellow, red or purple backgrounds. They are distracting and distort color perception markedly. A neutral grey would be far more suitable, and according to Williams (1984), "many scientific photographers advocate the use of mid-grey backgrounds for colored specimens."

Falsification of Perception of Colors Due to Colored Backgrounds

This has been attributed to:

1. The psychological process producing color tinging by transfer from the background to the subject (Blaker, 1977c).
2. Colored light from a transilluminated background reflected onto the specimen, adding a false hue to the specimen (Breckenridge and Halpert, 1953).

As Burgess (1975) points out, "there is some dispute as to how the surrounding colour influences the interpretation of the specimen with regards to the viewers' perception of hue and saturation." However, apart from colored light reflected from the background or originating from a transilluminated colored background, the change in color perception is more likely to be due to *color adaptation*. This has been succinctly described by Kodak (1972c) and is subdivided into three main types: (a) general color adaptation, (b) local color adaptation, and (c) lateral color adaptation. These operate simultaneously but are relatively independent of the adaptation to brightness. *General color adaptation* is the visual adaptive mechanism by which illumination tends to appear colorless, and thus caucasian skin is seen as the same color whether the illumination is by midday sun, by the reddish light of the setting sun or the yellowish-red light of tungsten bulbs. This effect, known as *approximate color constancy*, is due in large part to "remembering" colors rather than scrutinizing them.

Local color adaptation results in colored afterimages when the eye gazes fixedly at an area. Thus, if a yellow spot on a black background is viewed for 20 seconds, the retina becomes fatigued to that color, and when the gaze is transferred to white surface, an afterimage of the complementary color (blue in this case) appears on a white background.

Lateral color adaptation is similar in effect to *lateral brightness adaptation*, the visual effect by which the tone (grey value) of a subject appears different, depending on the tonal values of the surrounding area. Thus, a mid-grey area surrounded by white appears darker than the same mid-grey surrounded by black. The effect of *lateral color adaptation* is beautifully illustrated by Kodak (1972c) in four photographs of a blue patch surrounded by a white, black, yellowish-green and magenta rectangle. When surrounded by yellowish-green which is almost a complementary color, the patch appears more bluish. Thus, these findings indicate that adjacent complementary colors distort the perception of a color despite the attempt of color constancy to adjust the mental perception of that color to the approximate memory of it. However, problems arise in viewing a totally unknown subject, and here a neutral background (e.g. grey) allows the eye a reference point to "calibrate" itself. Thus, there can be little doubt that colored backgrounds do not allow the viewer an unbiased visual evaluation of pathological specimens.

Colored backgrounds are not always contraindicated; sometimes they have a desirable psychological effect when accuracy of color perception is not important. An example is projection of transparencies of formalin-fixed brain slices with a sky blue background for anatomical studies. The white brain slices with a blue background are reminiscent of a sky with clouds, and a whole series of these slides can be projected without viewers' fatigue. Also, the light reflected from the screen illuminates the room and adds to the feeling of brightness. This desirable psychological effect maintains viewers' interest. On the other hand, brain slices on a black background are psychologically depressing and visually tiring because of the high contrast, and these factors result in diminished viewers' interest.

GREY BACKGROUNDS

White backgrounds produce glare in projected transparencies, black backgrounds concentrate attention at the junction of the background and the specimen, colored backgrounds falsify perception of colors in the specimen; thus, the implication is that some tone of grey is the ideal background. Blaker (1977a) strongly opposes their use in monochrome prints, chiefly because of the difficulty in reproducing them accurately in printed material. Greys are usually darkened in printing and may be blotchy or uneven and consequently distracting in other than the highest quality printing. However, grey backgrounds have much to recommend them for transparencies. Unlike black, they do not concentrate the viewers' attention at the border of the specimen and background and do not result in a false perception of color. This raises the question, Why are they not used more extensively? Unfortunately, large uniformly grey backgrounds are difficult to obtain. Color casts caused by lighting, transilluminated glass, reciprocity failure, storage and processing of film are visible. Another major problem is that of obtaining repeatable results. Grey scale values depend on exposure. Even with standardized specimen lighting, exposure still has to be adjusted to allow for the reflectivity of the specimen. Bleached formalin-fixed brain slices require one-stop less exposure than fresh abdominal organs. Black pigmented skin requires an additional one-stop exposure. Thus, if the lighting intensity of the grey background is constant, the background in photographs of white brain slices will be darker because of reduced exposure, and lighter in photographs of black skin because of increased exposure. Attempts to compensate for this effect by controlling the lighting of the grey background or by varying the output of a transilluminated light box are very difficult and have not been completely successful. Controlling the lighting intensity of a transilluminated light box by a rheostat, which is the simplest method, alters color temperature, thus producing a color cast. Also, because of brightness adaptation, the human eye is not a very reliable judge of grey scale values (Marshall, 1957). The problem of how to achieve grey backgrounds of a constant tone value has yet to be solved.

An infinitely variable grey background is advantageous in monochrome photographs. The effect of differences in brightness of blue backgrounds and specimens has been investigated by Harris (1956) who recommended that if in doubt, a balanced background with the specimen and background having the same tonal values should be tried. If tonal contrast is desired, a background twice as dark or twice as light as the specimen should "yield pleasing results" (Harris, 1956). A balanced background results when the light from the transilluminated background equals that reflected from the specimen, the latter measured with the transilluminating lights off. However, Halsman (1955) has warned that backgrounds and specimens that match in luminance make the true shape and appearance of the specimen difficult to discern, although acuity in the specimen itself is aided. He considers it desirable to have the background tone slightly darker than that of the specimen, and to obtain this he recommends that the background have one-third stop less exposure than that required for the specimen. The rationale is that the darker background directs the viewers' eye into the lighter specimen. However, many of these dark grey backgrounds are psychologically somber, and a very light grey or white background is frequently preferred in monochrome photographs.

Disadvantages of Grey Backgrounds in Transparencies

These are:

1. Color casts are readily visible.
2. Shadows are frequently visible and are difficult to eliminate.
3. The tone of the grey background must be different than that of the edge of the specimen, otherwise the specimen and background will merge.
4. Large uniformly grey backgrounds are difficult to obtain.

Despite their well-recognized virtues, until some easy method of obtaining reproducible grey backgrounds is devised, their use with gross pathological specimens will continue to be limited. Comparison photographs of similar specimens should have grey backgrounds of the same tone. Obtaining identical backgrounds is difficult and time-consuming which is a problem when photographing delicate specimens which dry out quickly and lose their bloom.

Marshall (1957) found that when photographing radiographs and pathological specimens simultaneously by the method of Kent (1948), shadows of the specimen cast on the radiograph were of low contrast and poorly defined because of the radiograph's dense non-reflecting surface and were not reproduced in the photograph. Using a combination of different intensities of transillumination with radiographs of different densities, he produced background densities ranging from black through grey to white. There was one limitation. Shadows were still visible when radiographs of low opacity were used with low levels of brightness from the subilluminator.

Methods for Controlling the Tone of Grey Backgrounds

Methods used include (Marshall, 1957):

1. Fixed light output of top (specimen) lights but background lights reduced in intensity by:
   a. Neutral density filters, e.g. fogged radiograph film over the background illuminator.
   b. Rheostat control of the illuminator.
2. As in 1, except that separate exposures are given for the specimen and background, i.e. specimens are exposed without background lighting to give correct exposure for the specimen and then the background exposed to produce the desired density, with the speci-

men lighting turned off. Method 2 has been used by Halsman (1955). It is more suited for monochrome photographs taken by a large camera. The majority of 35mm cameras do not permit convenient double exposure, and also, absolute rigidity in the camera stand is essential to prevent the formation of overlapping images.

3. Polarizing the light from a transilluminated background. Marshall (1957) placed a Polaroid® sheet between glass to protect it and inserted it above the subilluminator (Fig. 2.3). An analyzer fitted over the camera lens was adjusted visually to obtain a background tone which produced suitable contrast between the subject and the background. Alternatively, the position of the analyzer was calculated mathematically from the angle of the polarizer and the transmission of the polarizer and analyzer. This method, although effective, has the disadvantage of the cost of large Polaroid® sheets for the light box and also precludes the use of polarized light to control specular highlights on specimens. The position of the analyzer which gives a suitable tone of background may not be the one which is optimal for the control of specular highlights.

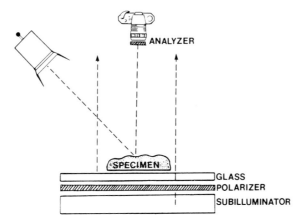

Figure 2.3. Variable grey background (Marshall, 1957). Light from the light box is polarized and then the depth of the grey tone of the background is adjusted by the polarizer (analyzer) on the camera. Courtesy of *Medical and Biological Illustration.*

LIGHT BOXES

In an attempt to obtain a background variable from white through grey to black and also colored in the limited space of an autopsy facility, numerous transilluminated light boxes have been described in the medical photography literature. Because of their importance, these will be reviewed below. However, it is advantageous to consider the features desired in such a box. These include:

1. Even illumination, no shadows or "hot spots."
2. Variability of tone from white through greys to black with no color casts.
3. Ability to introduce different colors, whose tone values can also be altered.

For practical use in the necropsy room, other desirable features include:

1. Easily changed backgrounds.
2. Easily controlled levels of illumination to allow standardization.
3. Color temperature of illuminator matched to that of the top (specimen) lights.
4. Easily cleaned and relatively waterproof.
5. Easily replaced glass top.
6. Adequate cooling of lights so that the specimen is not overheated and glass does not crack.
7. Adequate size to accept the majority of large specimens.
8. Relatively robust, e.g. glass not easily displaced and broken.

Theory of the Light Box

Hopes of obtaining a shadowless homogenous background with infinitely variable tone control from white through grey to black and with the option of adding color have attracted many to "light boxes," of which there are two main types:

1. *Transilluminated.* Lamps illuminate a diffuser, usually opalized glass or plastic placed below a glass plate supporting the specimen.
2. *Indirectly Illuminated.* Small lamps or fluorescent tubes on the side of the box shine on an opaque background underneath the plate glass supporting the specimen.

Both of these have different advantages and limitations and will be discussed separately.

1. **Transilluminated Light Boxes.** In these, the light source is diffused by

opalized glass (either single-flashed opalized glass, double-flashed opalized glass or solid opal glass) or, occasionally, ground glass. The actual light sources may already be partly diffused, e.g. from fluorescent tubes (Fig. 2.6). Design features such as baffles in the box, the proximity of tungsten lamps or fluorescent tubes to each other, number of lamps, reflectivity of the inside of the box, the distance from the lamps to the diffusing glass and the ability of the glass to diffuse, e.g. single opalized as compared to double opalized, all affect the evenness of the transilluminated light. The height of the diffusing glass above the light source is very important, and the best position for even diffusion can be determined by trial and error. The diffusing glass should be as close as possible to the light source and still achieve even illumination. This allows the distance between the specimen glass and the diffuser to be as large as possible so that shadows can be diffused and thrown out of the field of view of the lens.

Control of Shadows. There is a common misconception that shadows that fall on the opalized glass can be removed by "burning them out" by increasing the intensity of the transillumination. This is true if the ultimate objective is to obtain a completely clear white background. However, high levels of transillumination can result in flare into the camera lens with resultant degradation of the image. The usual requirement is not for a white background but for a homogenous light grey background. The only way to avoid differences in tonal values in the background is to prevent shadows from falling on the diffusing glass. Thus, the factors which determine whether or not shadows fall within the field of view have to be understood. From Figure 2.4 it is obvious that factors involved include:

1. Angle between the camera's optical axis and the lamp's axis.
2. Size of specimen.
3. Distance between the top clear specimen glass and the diffuser.
4. The angle of acceptance of the camera lens, a factor completely dependent on focal length.
5. Whether the beam of light is parallel or diffuse. Non-parallel light beams will produce larger, although less sharply defined, shadows.

Many lighting arrangements use one or more lamps at 45°. The diffusing glass will have to be positioned at twice the width of the specimen below the specimen support plate for the shadows to move the width of the specimens to the side, if the light source has parallel rays.

Thus, an object whose width is 7 inches will have its shadow cast the same distance to the side, if the glass is 7 inches below. This is no help in eliminating shadows from the field of view of a 50mm lens with a 45° acceptance angle, because the shadows will still be within the field of view. If a long focus lens with a narrower acceptance angle is used, shadows may fall outside the field of view of that lens (Fig. 2.4).

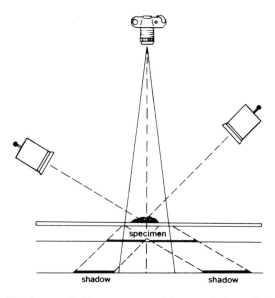

Figure 2.4. Effect of background distance on positions and sizes of shadows cast by two lamps at 45° and 60° lighting angles. As the background is lowered, the shadows are cast to the side.

Many of the designs of transilluminated and reflected light boxes have been reviewed by Martinsen (1952). One of the earliest described was by Harding (1933) cited by Martinsen (1952) which had two diffusers, a ground glass plate 6 inches below the top and a top opal glass (Fig. 2.5). Specimens were placed directly on the opal glass. Ground glass has the severe disadvantage of introducing a green color cast and thus is not suitable for color photography. Opal glass, which may be coated (flashed) on either one or two sides, is more suitable as a diffuser. Martinsen (1952) states that the ground-glass diffuser is not needed in the Harding box if the tungsten lamps are replaced by fluorescent tubes. A somewhat similar box has been described by Schaelow (1955) for botanical specimens. Again, the specimens were placed directly on ⅛ inch thick opal glass which lay on top of ¼ inch thick plate glass. Presumably, the ¼ inch plate glass gave strength to the ⅛ inch opal glass which was used because it was more economical than ¼ inch. However, both of these boxes have in common a top opalized glass on which visible shadows were cast by the specimen. To prevent that, later designs placed the flashed opal glass above the lamps to act as a diffuser, but well below the top ¼ inch plate glass which carried the specimen. There are other advantages to this second arrangement. Opalized glass is much more expensive than ¼ inch plate glass, and frequent cleaning eventually results in scratching of the opalizing. Also, shadows from the subject, instead of falling on the opal glass, now fall below and outside the field of view of the camera, if the subject is small enough and the specimen-diffuser distance is long enough, usually a couple of times the maximum dimension of the specimen.

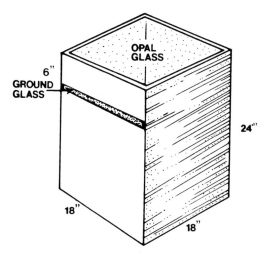

Figure 2.5. Harding light box with a ground glass diffuser and opal top glass. This arrangement gives excellent diffusion, but shadows cast by the specimen are visible on the opalized surface of the top glass.

Numerous variations in light box design are summarized in Tables I and II. The fact that Burgess (1975) states that "most workers will find it preferable to construct a transilluminator designed to their own specification" implies that few are totally satisfactory. This is partly true, but little attention has been given to the factors that limit the success of light boxes. A critical look at Table II will reveal that there is no consistency in the height of the specimen glass above the diffuser. The whole problem of a transilluminated light box for photography of large gross pathological specimens is an engineering problem that still needs to be solved. The authors' list of desirable features for such a hypothetical box for small pathological specimens is:

1. Maximum dimensions of top glass is 21 × 21 inches, for the same reasons given above for the black box.
2. Infinitely variable light output producing white through grey through black backgrounds.
3. Even illumination.
4. No change in color temperature with change in the intensity of the background illumination.
5. Color temperature identical to that of (top) specimen lights.
6. Option of adding colored backgrounds.
7. Shadowless for specimens up to a specified size, preferably up to 12 inches in diameter.
8. On smooth-running castors or steel rollers.

Table I
TRANSILLUMINATED LIGHT BOXES WITH FLASHED OPAL TOP GLASS

Author	Total Size *Length × Width × Height* *in Inches*	Diffuser	Top Glass	Lamps
Harding (1933)	18 × 19 × 24 high	ground glass 6 inches below top glass	opal glass	Unspecified number of incandescent bulbs bulbs
Schaelow (1955)	24 × 16 × 16 high (60 × 40 × 40cm)	none	⅛ inch opal glass supported directly on ¼ inch plate glass	6 × 200W incandescent bulbs
X-ray Illuminators	15 × 18	none	opal glass	fluorescent tubes

Fluorescent lamps are used in many light boxes because they require less diffusion to produce even illumination and their low profile allows the diffuser to be close to the lamps, thus keeping the specimen glass-diffuser distance as large as possible. Unfortunately, many of these boxes are, of necessity, rectangular to accept 40W (48 inches long) fluorescent tubes. These have the advantages of being available in a variety of color

Table II
TRANSILLUMINATED LIGHT BOXES WITH CLEAR TOP GLASS

Author	Total Size Length × Width × Height in Inches	Distance from Specimen Glass to Opal Glass in Inches	Distance from Opal Glass to Bottom of Box in Inches	Lamps
Beiter & Bohrod (1944)	18 × 16 × 12	5–7	5	not specified
Walters (1973)	30 × 22 × 12	5	7	20 × 40W lamps & 10 × 60W strip lamps
Burgess (1975)	30 × 20 × 18 approx.	12	6	3 fluorescent tubes
Halsman & Ishak (1977)	18 × 15 × 18	6	12	ringflash
Haeberlein (1979)	52 × 24 × 20 (130cm × 60cm × 50cm)	14 (35cm)	6 (15cm)	several fluorescent tubes in close contact with diffuser
Cornell University	30 × 24 × 20 + legs or castors	12	8	4 × 20W fluorescent tubes
Murdoch University	36 × 24 × 16	7	9	6 × 40W fluorescent tubes
Ontario Veterinary College, University of Guelph	48 × 30 × 22 + castors	15	8	6 × 40W fluorescent tubes
Purdue University	36 × 30 × 23	4	18	50W and 100W opal bulbs

temperatures and are capable of being dimmed. However, a 48 inch long light box is too long to fit conveniently between most specimen lamps, although the 48 × 30 inch light box at the University of Guelph is an outstanding exception (Table II, Figs. 2.6 and 2.7). The rectangular format unconsciously biases the photographer to place the specimen with its long dimension in the horizontal format, even if this is not its anatomically correct position during life. A square surface prevents this, but a 48 × 48 inch box would be unmanageable. A square box using 24 inch 20W fluorescent tubes could be built, but unfortunately fluorescent tubes of that length are not available in the variety that the 40W are and, at present, commercial dimmers for them are not available.

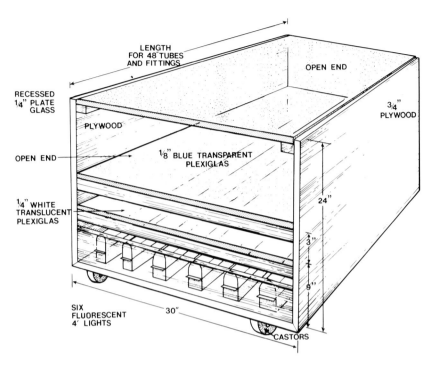

Figure 2.6. Transilluminated light box. The 48 × 30 inch box is illuminated by six fluorescent tubes diffused by a ¼ inch white translucent Plexiglas sheet. A ⅛ inch blue transparent Plexiglas may be added to the middle slot. Courtesy of the Department of Veterinary Pathology, Ontario Veterinary College, University of Guelph.

If a suitable light box were available to meet the above criteria, it would simplify gross specimen photography enormously. Colored backgrounds used nowadays, because they disguise uneven illumination, would be unnecessary.

2. **Indirectly Illuminated Light Boxes.** Dent (1937) devised a light box which could be used either as a transilluminated or a reflected light box (Fig. 2.8). Transillumination was achieved by placing it on top of the flashed opal glass of a transilluminated light box. For reflected light, opaque cardboard backgrounds were inserted into the housing. The apparatus was capable of producing backgrounds varying from white through various tones of grey to black. White and grey backgrounds were obtained by transillumination, with the light intensity being controlled by a rheostat. In the reflected-light mode, the intensity of the miniature top lamps in the box was adjusted to produce various tones of grey by light reflected from opaque grey backgrounds inserted into the

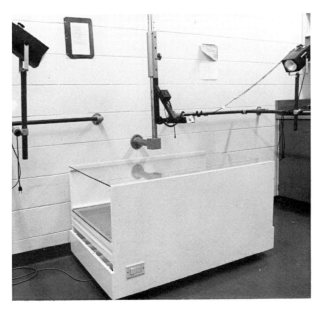

Figure 2.7. Ontario Veterinary College transilluminated light box and wall-mounted electronic flash units. Courtesy of Doctor Ian Wilkie.

box (Fig. 2.8). Dent (1937) emphasized illuminating the subject to its best advantage without considering the background and then adjusting the background tone to harmonize with the appearance of the subject and show it to its best advantage in monochrome photography. This takes some experience. Black velvet was used to produce an absolutely black background. The Dent box measured 14 × 7 inches overall but was capable of handling specimens only in the range of 1/10 inch to 7 inches. This fact points out one of the major difficulties with this type of box: the maximum size of the specimen is considerably smaller than the maximum size of the box. Dent (1937) emphasized that extraneous light from unused backgrounds should be controlled by masks, and that lamps in the top housing should be mounted at least 45° to the optical axis of the camera to prevent their light reflecting from the background directly into the lens. The Dent box gave excellent results with small dry specimens such as teeth and shells.

The principle of illuminating an opaque background in the Dent box has been used in larger boxes (Table III) for gross specimen photography (Fig. 2.9). To obtain maximally diffused light, 40W and 20W fluorescent tubes have been used. However, these boxes have suffered from the following faults:

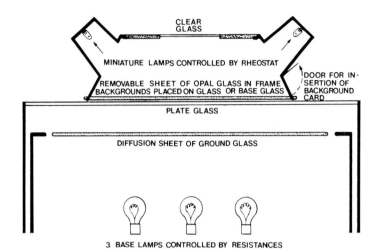

Figure 2.8. Dent box. The specimen is illuminated by miniature lamps in the box itself. The background can be transilluminated, from the light box below or can be opaque. Redrawn with permission from *British Journal of Photography.*

1. Uneven illumination of the background. The center of the background is physically distant from the light sources mounted around the periphery and thus receives less light.
2. The fluorescent lights cannot be varied in intensity.
3. The maximum specimen size is relatively small compared to the overall size of the box. A box 36 × 30 inches with a top glass of 30 × 24 inches has a utilizable opening of only 23 × 16 inches (Table III). However, because that opening is several inches below the top specimen glass, the largest specimen that can be accommodated is 18 × 12 inches with a 35mm camera used in a horizontal format and 12 × 9 inches in a vertical format. Thus, the largest specimen which a box whose outer dimensions are 36 × 30 inches (a very large box) can accommodate is 18 × 12 inches. This emphasizes the difficulty of developing a suitable light box for large specimens under a vertically mounted camera.
4. Fluorescent tubes of correct color temperature have not been available in 20W tubes to match the color temperature of the lamps used to illuminate the specimens. Kodak (1979) recommends "warm white deluxe fluorescent tubes for use with type A film, e.g. Kodachrome 40," although their light is not identical in color temperature with that of any specimen lights.

Table III
REFLECTIVELY ILLUMINATED LIGHT BOXES

	Total Size *Length × Width × Height in Inches*	Specimen *Glass Size in Inches*	Size of Area of Specimen *Glass Available for Specimen in Inches*	*Lights, Number & Type in Box*
Dent (1937)	14 × 7 × ?	8½ × 6½	8¼ × 6½	4 rows miniature incandescent bulbs; rheostat controlled
Whitley (1953)	19 × 19 height variable from 3–12 inches	14 × 14	. . .	4 × 60W strip lamps, independently switched
Smialowski and Currie (1958)	20 × 20 × 20	20 × 20	20 × 20	none—passively illuminated by 500W photofloods.
Ontario Veterinary College (1964)	30 × 28 × 14	20 × 18	less than 20 × 18	10 60W opal bulbs around periphery. One in each corner, one in middle of 28 inch side, 2 on 30 inch side
University of Melbourne (1964)	36 × 30 × 19	30 × 24	23 × 16	4 20W fluorescent tubes
University of Tennessee (1980)	24 × 21 × 20	36 × 21	24 × 21	none—passively illuminated by 2 Colortran Multi-6 650W lamps.
Texas A&M University (Hall, 1986)	60 × 34 × 30 modified desk	42 × 34	42 × 34	none—passively illuminated by 4 Colortran Mini-Pro 650W lamps.

5. The top glass has to be sealed into the box to prevent water dropping onto electrical circuits.

The advantage of a reflected light box is that backgrounds are easily changed in color and tone. Opaque backgrounds are merely inserted through a hatch. These may be cardboard from an art supply store or a variety of heavy paper backgrounds obtainable from the BD Company (2011 W. 12th Street, P. O. Box 3057, Erie, Pennsylvania 16512). However,

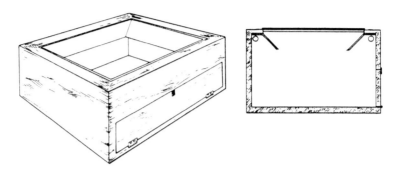

Figure 2.9. Large reflected light box (36 × 30 inches) which can accommodate an 18 × 12 inch specimen. Backgrounds are changed through the side door. The side elevation shows the fluorescent tubes and their light shields to reflect the light onto the opaque background.

tests have to be done because the color of many backgrounds records differently on film than as preceived by the eye.

3. **Passively Illuminated Light Boxes.** While transilluminated or reflected light boxes are excellent in theory, they work best for small specimens. In the necropsy room, relatively few of these boxes produce a consistent grey tone in sequential photographs because of changes in the number of top lights used or in changes in exposure made to compensate for specimen reflectivity. Background tones are difficult to match visually when some specimens are illuminated by one lamp and others by two. Some photographers are happy with their light boxes, but these usually have deeply saturated blue or green backgrounds with two or more standardized lights illuminating the specimen. Difficulty in maintaining background tone without color shift, obtaining uneven illumination and eliminating shadows has led to disillusionment with transilluminated light boxes. An alternative is the passively illuminated light box developed by Smialowski and Currie (1958) (Fig. 2.10). Ours has the following features:

1. Square top, specimen glass area is 21 × 21 inches.
2. Open ends and sides so that the background is illuminated by the same lamps that illuminate the specimen. Illumination is even if care is taken not to close the lower barn doors on the lamps.
3. The background is 21 × 24 inches. Its tone can be varied either by using interchangeable grey backgrounds of different tonal values or by raising or lowering this background towards or away from the specimen. We use several boards painted flat grey varying from light grey to dark grey and also white and black. Glossy surfaces

are unsuitable as they may reflect the top lights and cause gleaming highlights. The correct grey has to be found by trial and error. What appears as mid-grey to the eye may record on color film as dark grey, frequently with a color cast. Therefore, trial and error is necessary to find the correct color. A grey with the same tonal value as the Kodak Neutral Test card (18% reflectance) is a good initial starting point, although in most cases it will be too dark. Cardboard photographic backgrounds may be obtained from BD Company (2011 W. 12th Street, P.O. Box 3057, Erie, Pennsylvania 16512).

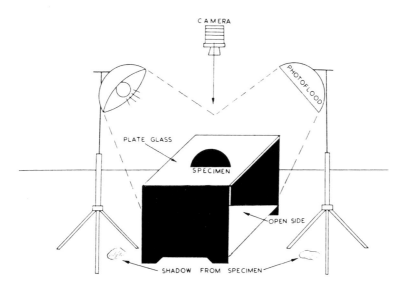

Figure 2.10. Passively illuminated light box. Reproduced with permission from Smialowski, A., and Curry, D. J., 1960, *Photography in Medicine.*

A passively illuminated light box was incorporated in an old desk by Hall (1986, Pers. Com.). The top glass plate was approximately 34 × 42 inches and backgrounds were 32 × 38 inch boards with colored or black velveteen stapled on both sides. These boards slid into slots 10, 15 and 22 inches below the specimen glass. Thus, backgrounds of different colors could be selected and the tone of the background could be changed by elevating or lowering the board. Lighting was supplied by 4 Color-tran Mino-Pro lamps—one at each corner of the desk top. To control the position and density of background shadows, lamps were raised or lowered or turned off until the background shadows were unobtrusive.

Thus, the basic technique was to adjust the lighting to control background shadows.

White backgrounds record as very light grey and are unsuitable to produce white backgrounds in monochrome photographs. Aluminum foil backgrounds have been used to produce very light grey backgrounds. Black painted wood reproduces as very dark grey, 8 or 9 on a 10-step grey scale. Black velvet remnants, which can be discarded if contaminated, can be used to obtain a totally black background. Unfortunately, when only one low-placed texture light at 80° to the camera's axis is used, the background may be unevenly illuminated. Photographs of brain slices taken with a black laminated plastic background look very good, because the background in the transparencies is very dark grey (tone values of 8 or 9 on a 10-step scale). These transparencies have less contrast between the brain and the background than the pure black background produced by a black box, and thus viewing these slides is less fatiguing.

Disadvantages of the passively illuminated reflected light boxes include:

1. Distracting shadows from the edges of the glass are cast across the middle of the visible background, particularly if non-diffused lights are used. Extending the glass approximately 8 inches beyond each end of the top of the box casts these shadows outside the field of view of the camera. A glass 36 inches long × 21 inches wide and 1/4 inch thick is used on a box whose supports are 21 × 21. The glass is heavy but not unwieldy.

2. If the front and back of the box are made of solid wood, then the option to rotate the box to select the best lighting angle for the specimen is precluded as the box's sides cast shadows across the background. One alternative is to have the glass supported only by thin corner steel posts which cast only minor shadows.

3. A pure white background for monochrome prints is not possible.

4. Large specimens cast shadows onto the background.

If the background is 20 inches below the glass, no shadows are cast by the left (60°) light, and acceptably diffused shadows are cast if both lights are used. However, if the right (45°) lamp alone is used, a prominent deep shadow is cast on the background. This cannot be avoided, but fortunately there are few cases where illumination by the right lamp alone is desirable. It is really a fill-in lamp for the 60° main light.

The maximum size of the field of view with the background board 24 inches below the top glass (21 × 21 inches) is 9 × 6 inches with a 35mm camera in a vertical format and 12 × 9 inches in a horizontal format. The effective size of the background can be increased markedly if the background is moved closer to the specimen. Thus, if the background is moved to 10 inches below the glass, the maximum size of specimen accommodated is 16 × 12 inches in a horizontal format and 12 × 9 inches in a vertical format for a 35mm camera. However, because the background is now closer to the specimen, there are prominent shadows from each lamp, whether used singly or together. This configuration, with the background close to the specimen glass, should be used only if the specimen is large and occupies most of the field of view thus obscuring the shadows. If the background shadows are distracting, the only alternative is to use the black box which will hold specimens up to 20 × 20 inches on a uniformly black background.

The inserted backgrounds measure 21 × 24 inches and are matte to prevent reflections. Easily cleaned matte plastic laminates are preferred. White, black, dark grey, grey with 18 percent reflectance (similar to that of the Kodak Neutral Test Card) and a light grey (approximately 36% reflectance) are used to vary the tone of the background. Thus, backgrounds have to be "calibrated" by trial and error. This includes selecting a background which records on film as the desired tone and color and determining the maximum size of specimen accommodated without casting shadows on the background when this is set at different distances below the specimen glass.

Specimen Glass. The top plate glass is usually ¼ inch thick and should be free of blemishes such as bubbles and scratches. Edges should be smoothed to prevent trauma to fingers. Specimens placed directly onto glass frequently ooze blood, exudate or edema fluid, and thus frequent cleaning of the glass is required. Obtaining a scrupulously clean glass is not easy, and smears are readily visible with oblique illumination from the specimen lights. The top glass should be easily removable so that it can be placed in a sink, washed thoroughly with hot water and detergent and then flushed with clean hot water. Glasses are wiped clean with *soft* disposable laboratory paper towels. The usual disposable paper towels will scratch glass. Scratches are a problem, because they are emphasized by texture lighting. Cleaning is necessary before each photography session. If glass is heavily soiled by a specimen, it is less effort to wash it with hot water and detergent in a sink than to try and clean it *in situ* by repeated wipings. If this is unsuccessful, stubborn smears can be removed by full strength "sudsy" ammonia or by Bon Ami®, which has been recommended as a non-abrasive cleaner for windshields (Pontiac, 1986). Sometimes one surface will be clean and the other streaked. To determine which side is streaked, wipe the two surfaces at right angles to each other. Debris such as glove powder or fine debris from the paper towels should be blown away by a judiciously directed blast of compressed air from a can. Smears should be removed by wiping with a soft towel after spraying lightly with a glass cleaner. This can be a commercial cleaner or made from the following formula recommended by Consumers Union (1980).

"Sudsy" ammonia	125ml
70% (isopropyl) alcohol	500ml
Liquid dishwasher detergent	7.5ml
Water to	4,000ml

Wet or moist smears are less visible than dried ones, which is another reason for expediting photography.

Disadvantages of Light Boxes of all Types

1. **Dirt and Smears of Blood and Exudate on the Glass.** These are highly visible. They can be difficult and time consuming to remove, particularly with specimens that continue to ooze blood or fluid.

2. **Reflections.** A glass plate supporting a specimen reflects anything above it, the camera, photographic stand, photographer, ceilings, lights and even the elevated portions of the specimen and the back of the rulers. Painting the camera stand black and using a black body camera is not adequate, as a black camera has gleaming corners and some chromed areas. The ceiling should be painted flat black. Overhead lights should be located so as not to reflect in the glass. This means positioning them several feet to the side and perhaps masking them with black shields. Reflections of the ruler can be controlled by blackening the back and sides of the ruler (see "Ruler"). However, reflections of the camera and stand are most easily prevented by a black reflection control plate made of stiff cardboard or metal plate positioned below the camera and with a hole sufficiently large to allow the lens to view the specimen. This plate can be mounted to the camera stand, or commercial models that screw into the lens filter mount are available. The latter type has the advantage of always being correctly positioned and is the only alternative if a camera's format can be changed from horizontal to vertical. Many camera shields are too small for large fields of view, and yet, with very small fields, as for example at RR = 1:2, they may obstruct lighting of the specimen. Some commercial shields have sides angled up at 20° to 45°,

but the angled sides may obstruct hand focusing of the lens. Alteration of this angle by trial and error may be necessary. The side of the shield towards the 45° lamp can be horizontal and the other side towards the 60° lamp can be bent upwards at 20° to 30° (Figs. 3.6 and 3.7). This arrangment allows easy focusing without the shield obstructing the lighting of the specimen.

3. **Uneven Illumination.** Many of the different designs do not give even illumination. Use of double-flashed opal glass instead of single-flashed; numerous small bulbs instead of a lesser number of larger bulbs; and increasing the distance between the bulbs and the diffusers all reduce uneven illumination in transilluminated light boxes. The reflected light box has great difficulty in supplying sufficient illumination to the center of the field, and thus there is a uniform falloff in illumination from the edges to the center.

4. **Inadequate Control of Brightness.** Excessively bright backgrounds cause flare and obscure the contours of the specimen (Haeberlein, 1979). Control of the brightness of tungsten lamps is relatively easy by using rheostats or dimmers, but there are no dimmers currently available commercially for small (24 inch) fluorescent tubes, and the ones for large (48 inch) tubes frequently cause flicker. Dimming causes change in color temperature in tungsten lamps.

5. **Colored Backgrounds.** These are usually highly saturated in an attempt to disguise uneven illumination.

6. **Excessive Heat.** This can break glass or dry out fluids on the glass, causing visible smears.

OPAQUE BACKGROUNDS

A wide variety of backgrounds including disposable paper, cardboard, surgical drapes and towels as well as painted wood and laminated plastic on wood and white enamel trays (Levin, 1939) have been used as opaque backgrounds. They have the advantage of simplicity but have serious deficiencies, including visible surface imperfections and obvious cast shadows. Hansell and Ollerenshaw (1962) claim that shadows cast by a subject increase the illusion of added depth. An isolated shadow on a dark background may be acceptable, but complex lighting produces multiple shadows that are distracting (Marshall, 1957). These are even more distracting if shadows from adjacent objects overlap, producing shadows of different densities and with colored backgrounds, shadows of different color saturations. Multiple shadows should be avoided at all costs (Haeberlein. 1979). Vetter (1969) states, "There should be only one shadow on a background and shadows should fall downward." If the shadow is in any other direction, the viewer may be confused and think the specimen is upside down.

Haber (1980) recommends "tray liners." These are disposable paper sheets used to cover the bottom of food trays and are available from the dietary department of hospitals. They are inexpensive, disposable and available in different colors and sizes. Dark blue is the most frequently used by Haber (1980) because shadows do not show. The thin paper liners are placed on glass elevated 6 to 8 inches above the baseboard and then illuminated from below by a slave flashgun to reduce shadows (Haber, 1982). Paper and cardboard backgrounds are unsuitable for wet specimens, because the paper becomes soggy and changes color and tone. Burgess (1975) recommends a matte-surfaced, plastic-coated background. We use plywood covered by a plastic laminate. Because of exposure to water and aqueous disinfectants, marine-grade plywood which is resistant to water is required. As black and transilluminated boxes produce successful backgrounds with most small specimens, use of opaque backgrounds is confined chiefly to large specimens and small cadavers. Our boards are 36 × 24 inches and will hold canine cadavers weighing up to 70 pounds. Plastic laminate (e.g. Formica®) is available in a variety of colors. We have tried light grey, green, bluish-green, white and black, all with a matte surface. Exactly how the color records on film cannot be predicted, and trials are recommended. A convenient way to do this is to photograph a finger placed on a sample "chip" (Fig. 2.11). Many dark grey plastic laminates record on film as browns rather than grey. Specimens on all opaque backgrounds except black have distracting shadows. A black Formica, "Angola brown #947-85, suede finish," has been the most successful opaque background. It records as a very dark brown on film, and shadows are not obvious. Dark grey laminates show objectionable shadows. Uneven illumination of the background is a frequent problem with flash photography. Plastic laminates produce specular reflections if they have been cleaned with a spray polish which produces a glossy surface. Cleaning with mild scouring powder and water prevents this. Reflections of lamps from the background should be checked through the viewfinder.

We use a variety of different-sized boards as backgrounds for small cadavers and for flash photography of portions of large animals. Plastic

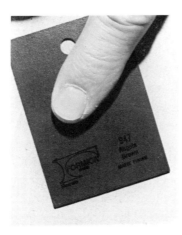

Figure 2.11. A simple method of checking the suitability of a plastic laminate as a background is to photograph a finger on a sample chip.

laminated boards have the disadvantages of cost and weight. The initial cost is moderately high, as marine-grade plywood is necessary because of exposure to water, but these backgrounds last for decades. Also, 1/2 inch or 3/8 inch thick boards are very heavy. A determining factor in their size is the width of the door to the photography room. The door opening should be at least 32 inches (and preferably 34 or 36 inches) to allow easy ingress of small animal cadavers carried on boards. Previous to employing plastic-laminated covered boards, we used painted boards. These have the disadvanges of a distinct surface texture and of requiring frequent repainting because of staining by blood and exudates.

Green surgical towels and drapes are favored by surgeons as a background. Burgess (1975) recommends a green theater (surgical) towel dampened in water. In our experience, they are very distracting because of both their texture and color. The weave of the cloth is particularly obtrusive with texture lighting (Fig. 2.12), and as Kodak (1972b) states, "The subject, rather than its surroundings, should exhibit the more noticeable texture." Disposable "tray liners" or plastic-laminated boards are preferred. We have tried Teflon®-coated "cookie sheets." They were easy to clean, had matte surfaces and no texture, but most of the colors were unsuitable as photographic backgrounds.

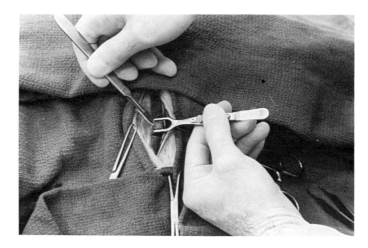

Figure 2.12. Surgical towel. Note the obtrusive texture.

Backgrounds for Flash Photography

Flash illumination in the necropsy room is usually confined to photographs of whole large animals or their organs *in situ*. Backgrounds present a real difficulty. Stainless steel tables are undesirable, as they may reflect light from the flash unit into the camera or record as almost black. We use 34 × 36 inch black plastic laminate covered plywood boards. Results are excellent, provided that the flash head is not mounted directly on the camera so that the flash is reflected off the board into the lens. Thus, the flash head needs to be held above and to the side where it also gives better modeling. If the flash cannot be angled to prevent reflections, an alternative is to tilt the background. However, the flash sensor must be mounted on or be incorporated in the camera to ensure accurate exposure if automatic exposure is used. Colored backgrounds have been tried for this type of photography but are distracting. The black plastic laminate, Formica Angola brown #947-85, suede finish, is suitable, as even very dark specimens do not merge with it.

The advantages of opaque backgrounds such as plastic laminated covered plywood are that they are robust, easy to clean, and ooze from specimen is not as obvious or as difficult to clean as on glass. However, these backgrounds are inflexible, and cast shadows can be obtrusive. They are most useful as backgrounds for small animals and portions of large animals, particularly when the amount of background included in the photograph is minimized.

SUMMARY

In gross specimen photography, black, grey and white backgrounds are required. Currently, there is no single piece of equipment which can provide backgrounds in tones from white to black for large specimens in the necropsy room. Several pieces of equipment are required. We use a black box (specimen glass 21 × 21 inches) to obtain a black background for specimens where the outline must be emphasized, a reflected light box with a specimen glass of 21 × 21 inches to obtain grey backgrounds, and an illuminated rheostat-controlled light box (specimen glass 21 × 21 inches) for light grey or white backgrounds, chiefly for monochrome photography. Also, opaque plywood backgrounds 36 × 24 inches covered by black Formica "Angola brown" #947-85 suede finish are used for large specimens, small cadavers and specimens that continue to ooze blood or serum.

All of these backgrounds have disadvantages and advantages, both photographically and in the presentation of the specimen. Generally, monochrome prints need white or light grey backgrounds, and so a transilluminated light box is essential. For color transparencies, grey backgrounds are best, but maintaining the same tone value from photograph to photograph is difficult to achieve. To emphasize the outline of light-toned specimens, a black background is best. Where accuracy of color perception is not important, blue or bluish-green backgrounds are psychologically and visually pleasing.

RULERS

An indicator of size is necessary in every photograph, especially in veterinary pathology where there is such great variation in the size of normal organs among different animals. In the past, a variety of objects including hands, fingers, thumbs, pencils, pens, cigarettes, coins, matches, matchboxes, scalpels, artery forceps (hemostats), thimbles, walnuts, peanuts, eggs, nails, pins, screws, keys and rulers graduated in inches have all been used in scientific photography (Kent, 1947; Halsman, 1955; Smialowski and Currie, 1960a; Martin, 1961). As Martin (1961) points out, "the presence of a half-crown (a now discontinued coin) reposing on the wall of a dilated colon is repugnant." The most suitable indicator of measurement is a centimeter ruler, although this has limited accuracy, because only the plane of the specimen at the level of the principal plane of focus will be at the same scale in photographs of specimens of significant depth (Martin, 1961). Like the background, the ruler should be unobtrusive so that attention is not diverted from the specimen (Carl, 1980). Selection of a suitable ruler would appear to be relatively simple, but there are few, if any, commercially available rulers suitable for scientific photography. This explains the numerous recommendations on how to produce suitable rulers photographically (Haeberlein, 1979; Martin, 1961; and Martinsen, 1968).

Location

Halsman (1955) recommends that the "rulers be placed at the edge of the field and held to a practical minimum size." The ruler should also be placed at the anatomic bottom of the specimen (Fig. 2.13) (Halsman, 1955; Vetter, 1969; Martin, 1961; Burgess, 1975) where it is less obtrusive (Martin, 1961) and can be used to orient the viewer (Halsman, 1955). Another advantage of this position is that shadows from the ruler are not cast onto the specimen or background. The bottom position is not universally used (Hansell, 1946), but rulers at the top seem unnatural, and ones at the sides cannot be read easily and frequently cast shadows onto the specimen or background.

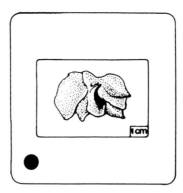

Figure 2.13. A centimeter ruler is placed in the lower right corner and kept to an unobtrusive minimum.

The ruler should neither touch nor be superimposed upon the specimen (Halsman, 1955). There are occasions when the ruler can be placed on top of the specimen; for example, in close-up photographs of gastric ulcers, the ruler can be inserted unobtrusively at the bottom right of the frame, on top of the gastric mucosa. Because some journals do not accept rulers in prints and others want them replaced by either a 1cm scale bar or a standardized scale inserted by the printer, it must be possible to remove the ruler without marring the photograph fo the specimen.

The problem of the use of rulers has been summarized by Sacco (1982), who states:

> My own practice is to add a ruler, but position it at the extreme edge of the negative or slide. This way it is a permanent part of the photo-graphic record, but it is far enough away from the subject that it can be cropped out and replaced by a verbal indication of size in the caption or by an unobtrusive scale bar in the picture itself. The key word here is "unobtrusive." A ruler interferes with the important image too much. A scale bar interferes less . . . [and] in the interest of appealing, unclut-tered photographs, a scale bar is preferable. It can be applied to the print with press-on transfer material (cut to length before applying) or drawn on with a drafting pen (which will write on glossy prints, contrary to popular belief).

Elevation of Ruler

The ruler should be in the plane of principal focus (Martin, 1961), and its surface should be parallel to that of the film plane to prevent distor-tion (keystoning). Recommendations to elevate the ruler to this plane have included the use of corks, copper tubing (Vetter, 1969), brass cylinders, matchboxes, film boxes, black and wooden blocks ($1 \times 3 \times 1$, $1 \times 3 \times 2$, $1 \times 3 \times 4$ inches) (Anon., 1942), pipette holders, a modified laboratory stand (Halsman and Ishak, 1977), and even special stands (Harp, 1965; Geddes, 1980). In our experience, modeling clay (plasticine) is the easi-est to use. Height and location can be adjusted easily by compressing and sliding the clay while viewing the specimen and ruler through the viewfinder.

If the specimen is large and a relatively short focal length lens is used, the material supporting the ruler may be visible. However, modeling clay can be placed outside the field of view and the ruler stuck to it so that it can project to the side into the desired position. Also, when a portion of an organ (e.g. stomach) is being photographed, one end of the ruler can lie on top of gastric mucosa while the other end is supported by modeling clay. Modeling clay is so cheap that it can be discarded or autoclaved when it becomes contaminated. The special scale holder (Harp, 1965) and laboratory stand (Halsman and Ishak, 1977) can be used only with smaller specimens because they occupy significant portions of the background. The stand designed by Geddes (1980) does not have this disadvantage, but it has to be glued to the specimen table. The major drawback to these stands is the risk of contamination. Special scale holders may be useful for non-pathological or fixed specimens, but in necropsy room photography, where contamination from gloves, specimens or backgrounds is likely, their disadvantages outweigh advantages. Disposable supports such as modeling clay and wooden blocks are more appropriate. Modeling clay has the disadvantage that it clings to the ruler, and while remnants of it may not be obvious to the naked eye, they will be very visible in macrophotographs. Dark-grey modeling clay is our choice. If it inadvertently becomes visible in the field of view, it is not obvious on black or grey backgrounds.

Length and Size of Ruler

For maximum usefulness, the ruler should extend the full width of the specimen (Harrison, 1950), or the full width of the frame, so that the size of the lesion or specimen can be determined easily. Carl (1980) recommends that the scale be at least half the length to slightly longer than the specimen or lesion. However, this may result in the ruler being very obtrusive. Martin (1961) recommends a "short segment." Some laboratories place a 1cm ruler in the middle of the bottom edge of the frame. This is also obtrusive. If the primary objective of the photograph is to record dimensions, then the ruler should be placed across the full length of the bottom of the frame. The ruler used should start at zero (Martin, 1961), and this zero graduation should be as close as possible to the left end of the ruler. Rulers which extend several mm to the left of zero should have this extra length machined off. Halsman (1955) recommends 3cm, 6cm and 12cm rulers for human specimens. In the absence of a supply of suitably sized rulers, we adjust the position of a ruler to a "practical minimum" (Halsman, 1955) by exposing 1cm of the ruler in the bottom right-hand corner of the frame and then sliding the ruler up or down to control the length of graduations visible in the field of view (Fig. 2.13).

Specifications of Rulers

1. **Rigidity.** Rulers are frequently supported in the middle and with the free end projecting into the field of view in the principal plane of focus. A non-rigid ruler is likely to bend.

2. **Flatness.** Many commercial rulers have sloping or beveled edges. As the plane of the graduations must be parallel to the film plane, such rulers have to be tilted. Unfortunately, suitable rigid flat rulers are rare.

3. **Texture.** To be unobtrusive, the ruler must be textureless but with a dull finish to prevent reflections. Wooden rulers are unacceptable because of both grain and texture (Martin, 1961). Plastic rulers are the most suitable, but any scratches will cause changes in texture and the ruler should be discarded. Stainless steel is unsuitable because it either reflects light or appears very dark when illuminated by raw (i.e. undiffused) light.

4. **Graduations.** Often, graduations are depressions filled with paint and are really changes in texture. They have the unfortunate ability to reflect small specular highlights resulting in degradation of the blackness of the line. These highlights are distracting, particularly in extreme close-ups. Black lines painted on the surface would be better, although they may be easily damaged as the ruler is cleaned. The zero graduation line should be only 0.5–1mm from the end. Graduations need to be fine, delicate and impeccably finished in rulers that will be highly magnified in close-up photographs. Graduations should be broad and bold and only at 0.5cm and 1cm lines in rulers of 25cm, 50cm or 1 meter length. Most commercial rulers are not designed for photography and thus do not meet these requirements. The direction of the lines strongly influences the obtrusiveness of the ruler. Only vertical calibrations are necessary, and horizontal lines are distracting and non-contributory. If the horizontal line is above the graduations, then the eye is deflected along it before it views the graduations. If graduations are placed along the bottom of the ruler and the ruler is placed along the bottom of the frame, the whole bulk of the ruler has to be included in the frame and cannot be "kept to the practical minimum" (Halsman, 1955). Only rulers with the graduations on top should be used.

5. **Size.** If a single size of ruler is used for specimens of all sizes, it will occupy a disportionately high percentage of the field of view of very small specimens, while it may be so small as to be illegible with large specimens. Numbered graduations need to be legible but unobstrusive. The relationship between legibility of numbers in a projected transparency and their size on the ruler has been investigated by Carl (1980). He found that the height of a number should not be smaller than 1/30th the height of the photographic frame if the number is to be legible when the projected image on the screen is viewed from a distance of 8 times the

height of the projected image. This viewing distance is usually considered the maximum screen-viewer distance and represents the outer limit of legibility. Carl also found that if the numbers were over 1/15th the height of the frame, they were too large and thus distracting. On the basis of these findings, he devised 4 different sized rulers for photographic fields ranging from 1 cm to 30 cm in length. Although the concept is excellent it has certain problems. To be unobtrusive, rulers should match the color and tone of the background. Therefore not only is the supply of different sized rulers required, but also different colored ones. Also numbers on the rulers are very distracting. Our policy is to use a *numbered* ruler only when actual measurements are of paramount importance or if the ruler is to be included in a negative and later replaced by a scale bar on the photographic print. To avoid the necessity of having a wide array of different sized rulers in different colors, we use rulers with no numbers and the size of the ruler in the photograph is controlled by moving it up or down to reveal an appropriate length of the graduations.

6. **Color and Tone.** To be unobtrusive, the ruler must be the same color as the background. This is easily accomplished with light backgrounds, particularly transilluminated ones, by using a transparent ruler with black graduations (Rogers, 1976; Fritts, 1976). The ruler must be perfect, as any blemishes such as scratches or defective graduations will be emphasized. However, for dark backgrounds, matching tone and color can be difficult or impossible to achieve, but an exact match is seldom needed for the ruler to be relatively unobtrusive. Thus, a black ruler with light grey vertical graduations is suitable for black and very dark grey backgrounds, and a light-toned ruler with black graduations is suitable for opaque light backgrounds such as light and mid-grey. However, a white or very light-toned ruler should be avoided (Anon., 1942), because it may produce a glaring highlight and possibly flare if extra exposure has been given to a dark specimen and has resulted in overexposure of the ruler. This is a common problem with disposable adhesive white labels. We use a light tan ruler with black graduations, but ivory, buff or light grey are suitable. In fact, if the ruler occupies only a small percentage of the frame, a light brown ruler with black graduations can be used with white or grey backgrounds, but for optimal results, the color (hue) and tone of the ruler and backgrounds should be similar. Thus, we use a black ruler on a black background and a dark grey on grey backgrounds. Both these rulers have light grey graduations,

not white lines which can be very glaring and distracting, particularly if longer than average exposures are required for dark specimens. We have been unable to locate commercial rulers that meet all of these specifications, but a tan New Math Ruler (Sterling Plastics Co., Mountainside, New Jersey 07092) is acceptable. Unfortunately, graduations start about 1cm from the end and this extra length has to be sawn off and the end smoothed in a machine shop. The ruler is also beveled and has to be tilted to place the graduations parallel to the film plane. However, these rulers are adequate and cheap enough to be discarded if contaminated or when graduations become marred.

7. **Lettering.** Many rulers sold by scientific supply houses advertise the name of the company. This makes them unsuitable for photography. Personally, we avoid all lettering on rulers, but Halsman (1955) recommends that the name of the institution be placed on the lower edge of the ruler. While no doubt, this may bring some honor to that institution, it, like all lettering and figures, distracts the viewer's attention. Such labeling is to be avoided unless the institution is attempting to retain copyright. A supply of different-sized rulers with different-sized names is required, otherwise the name may be excessively large with small specimens or illegible with large specimens.

Photographically Reproduced Rulers

Because of the dearth of suitable commercial rulers (Carl, 1980), there are papers describing how to produce suitable ones photographically (Halsman, 1955) (1) on clear 35mm film attached to Plexiglas (Martin, 1961), (2) on lithographic film (Rogers, 1976; Haeberlein, 1979) and (3) as prints mounted on cardboard (Martin, 1961; Martinsen, 1968; Rogers, 1976). Our own rulers for use with a black background are made by photographing a printed ruler with long centimeter and short millimeter graduations using a high contrast film. This is reversed. To avoid distracting stark white lines, graduations are printed light grey on a black background (Fig. 2.14). The photographic paper is matte to reduce reflections. Prints are dry mounted onto mounting board and trimmed to approximately 2cm wide and several cm long. The left-hand margin is cut approximately 1mm from the start of the ruler. The width of 2cm is sufficient to allow the photographer to manipulate the ruler without contaminating the graduations with modeling clay or fluids. As these rulers reflect in the glass holding the specimen, the back and all edges are blackened with a black felt-tipped marker pen. The ruler depicted in

Specimen Dissection and Photography

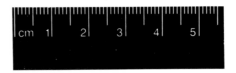

Figure 2.14. Photographically reproduced ruler for use with black and dark grey backgrounds. The graduations are light grey to prevent glare.

Figure 2.13 is suitable for RR = 1:2 up to RR = 1:10 by moving the ruler in and out of the field of view to include a length of graduations appropriate to the proportions of the frame.

Rulers for Black-and-White Prints

Prints are usually cropped for a variety of reasons such as to improve composition, to fit them into a page or column of a book or journal, or to form part of a composite plate. A ruler whose size and position were appropriate for the original print may now have an aesthetic defect such as being too large, not starting at 0 or being too far from the specimen. In other words, the proportions of the ruler, specimen and background have been changed. This is frequently disappointing, considering the effort made to balance these at the time the black-and-white negative was taken. The easiest solution is to remove the ruler from the print and to insert a 1cm scale bar, either a black line on a white background or a white line on a black background. This can be press-on transfer material cut to length or a line drawn by a drafting pen to the same scale as the ruler in the photograph (Sacco, 1982). Thus, the time and effort taken to insert a ruler in the field of view for monochrome photography is not warranted. The best solution is to place the ruler clear of the specimen in the principal plane of focus and along the bottom edge of the negative where it is part of the permanent record but can be cropped easily (Sacco 1982). There is another reason for not including the ruler in the final print. Because black-and-white prints are scrutinized so closely, even minor defects in the rulers themselves are much more evident than they are in projected 2 × 2 slides.

Defects in positioning rulers in gross specimen photographs are frequent in published articles. One prominent textbook of pathology had the following errors in positioning rulers: ruler not parallel to the bottom of the frame; on the side of the frame; tilted and not parallel to the film plane; across a whole frame but starting at 13, not 0; superimposed on the specimen; touching the specimen; between two specimens;

partially obscured by an overlapping specimen; ruler cast shadow on the specimen; specimen cast shadow on the ruler; and modeling clay visible under ruler. In the same book, defects in rulers themselves included: 15cm ruler under a 30cm long specimen; numbers at the top of the ruler and graduations along the bottom edge; buckled; 1mm graduations too small for large specimens; black ruler with white horizontal line along the top and graduations along the bottom; black ruler with numerous scratches and blemishes; graduations in inches not centimeters; and remnants of modeling clay on top of ruler. These findings emphasize the desirability of replacing rulers in prints with scale bars which are scientifically correct and aesthetically pleasing (Sacco, 1982).

Summary

A range of rulers of different sizes whose tone and color match those of the backgrounds and whose size is sufficient to produce legible images but still be unobtrusive is required for photography of gross specimens. Desirable features include rigidity, lack of texture (plastic), flatness (not beveled), unetched graduations, matte surfaces, absolutely straight edges and only 1mm extra length on the left end. Rulers should be available in various lengths and widths with fine graduation on small rulers and thick bold ones on large rulers. They should also be made in a variety of colors or grey tones, at least black with light grey graduations and tan, light grey or mid-grey with black graduations. Graduations should be vertical only, as a horizontal line is unnecessary and distracts attention. At present, suitable rulers for gross specimen photography are difficult to find, and a ruler that meets these criteria is prized and jealously guarded by the photographer. A supply of rulers meeting the above specifications and cheap enough to be discarded when contaminated or marred would considerably simplify color photography of gross specimens. A ruler in a print is best replaced by a scale bar, but a ruler should be included in the negative as part of the permanent record.

Identification Labels

Keeping an accurate record of specimens photographed is not difficult, particularly if only one case is recorded on each roll of film or at each job. To avoid any ambiguity, many necropsy laboratories place small labels bearing the accession number adjacent to, or even on, the specimen. There is considerable controversy as to the desirability of this practice.

The human eye is irresistably drawn to letters and numbers, and thus numbered labels, sometimes embellished with the name of the institution or even its crest, distract the viewers' attention from the specimen. However, such labels accurately identify specimens.

Label Should Be Used:

1. in monochrome and color negatives where a label can be masked or trimmed off the final prints but identifies the negative accurately.
2. when very large numbers of specimens from different cases are photographed on the same roll of film.
3. in legal cases where correct identification is of paramount importance.
4. in research trials such as a carcinogen trial with laboratory animals where photographs become part of the documentation and legal record.
5. in sequential photographs of the same clinical lesion over a period of weeks to years, e.g. a limbal plaque progressing to ocular squamous cell carcinoma on a bovine eye.

Disadvantages of Identification Labels

The major disadvantages are that they distract the attention of the viewer from the subject. They also reduce the amount of the frame available for the specimen. The latter point is particularly significant when photographing very small lesions, for there is a limit to the minimal size of a label.

An easy solution to these competing views is to take a series of two or more transparencies, the first frame with a label, the others without a label (Haber, 1980). Vetter (1960) uses the first frame of each roll of film to record the roll number, date, and name of the hospital. Details of individual frames are recorded on photographic request slips. In our necropsy laboratory, we use labels only in legal cases. For routine specimens, two or three frames are taken of every specimen and exposures recorded in the log book (see "Records"). On return from the processing laboratory, transparencies are matched with the records. Unidentified or incorrectly identified transparencies are a rarity.

Type of Label

Labels that have been used include: handwritten, typed paper or label-writer tape (Halsman and Ishak, 1977). All of these are distracting, particularly at high magnifications where imperfections are obvious. Also, labels are usually of one size and are thus barely legible in photographs of large fields and disportionately large when the ratio of reproduction approaches one-half. Labels are even more distracting if their color is different from that of the background. Labels should be made of rigid cardboard, the same color as the background and in the smallest size that is still legible. As the ruler occupies the bottom right-hand corner of the frame, we place the few labels we use in the bottom left at the same height as the ruler. Here, they can be masked off if necessary.

Halsman and Ishak (1977) placed their identification label on the ruler below the graduations. It is masked off in slides for projection. However, anything that widens the extent of the ruler in the field of view increases the "practical minimum size" (Halsman, 1955) and interferes with the proportioning and the composition. In other words, rulers and labels can become too large and obvious.

Labels in Legal Cases

We have no hesitation in using labels recording all pertinent data such as species, dates and other circumstances in the specimens when there is a possibility of legal action. Again we follow the policy recommended above of taking some with the label and some without. When large labels are removed, reframing, adjustment of the composition and refocusing may be necessary.

Speed and accuracy of photography have been emphasized above. The production of neat labels frequently is time consuming, especially when these have to be typed elsewhere and then the paper or cardboard trimmed. Because of the possibility of contamination by infectious material, typewriters should not be kept in the gross specimen photography room. Our policy is to use as few labels as possible and, when necessary (e.g. for legal purposes), use hand-lettered labels placed in the lower left corner. Such labels are made of cream or light-brown colored cardboard. White is to be avoided, because it is extremely distracting and produces glare as described above for white rulers. Accession numbers that bear the date have an adverse psychological effect on the interest of students, particularly when they calculate that the photograph was taken before they were born. Accurate identification, except in legal cases, can be maintained by omitting the year number from the label (e.g. 251 instead 85-251) and recording full details in a log book. Labels with complicated identification codes such as "SP-25 Z-6 Lit 2" are more likely to pique the interest of the viewer whose time will then be spent trying to decipher the code, rather than viewing the specimen.

Whether or not to include identification labels and rulers in prints provokes strongly held opinions. The best alternative is to include them in all negatives but to position them so that they can be excluded from the final print. In transparencies, rulers should be held to a practical minimal size and labels either omitted or placed where they can be masked off.

Pointers

These, like labels, are distracting. Needles, arrows cut from paper, pencils and pointing fingers have all been used to indicate anatomic structures or lesions on specimens (Halsman 1955). Pointers should be avoided, as they are liable to soiling, are notoriously difficult to attach in proper orientation (Martin, 1961), and, as Halsman (1955) also succinctly states, "the photographer has enough worry to compose a photograph without having to concern himself with arranging the height and direction of arrows." If it is decided to use arrows, these have to be of a size and color to be obvious without being distracting. Probably dark grey and mid-grey are least objectionable, but the major task is in the positioning. The arrows should lead the eye into the photograph, not out. Unfortunately, after taking care to position the arrows for good composition, cropping of the final print may result in labels being badly placed. Unfortunately, such arrows cannot be removed and, hence, it is far better to add arrows to the final print. Here, design and orientation can be easily controlled, and the results are superior to attaching arrows to the specimen itself. If anatomic structures or lesions are difficult to identify in a photograph and accurate identification is required, one frame can be taken using labels and then several without and labels added to the prints or transparencies later.

Specimens should be so dissected that salient features are evident without the need for pointers (Halsman, 1955), but even the best dissections may not indicate communicating defects from one cavity or lumen to another in a still photograph. Thus, in illustrating congenital septal defects in the heart, a probe may be necessary. Applicator sticks, scapel handles, knives, forceps, fingers, silver probes, colored bristles, rubber tubing and variously colored nylon threads have all been used. A suitable probe should not be distracting, and contrasting gaudy colors are unsuitable. Wooden applicator sticks are undesirable for the same reason as wooden rulers (i.e., grain, texture and even fine splinters). Stainless steel can record as almost black when illuminated by raw (undiffused) light and thus scapel handles and probes are unsuitable. Natural rubber cylinders such as urinary catheters are relatively unobtrusive in the same way as natural rubber gloves are. These catheters are also available in a variety of diameters, are flexible and can be cut to suitable lengths. We keep a supply of these in our photography room for use as probes.

Chapter 3

PHOTOGRAPHIC TECHNIQUE

LIGHTING

Haeberlein (1979) states that although there is no fundamental rule for the location of lamps for illuminating a specimen, the aim should be to produce "a natural type of lighting." To do this the subject must be oriented so that the light appears to come approximately from the top (Kodak, 1970), either from directly above or from the top left or right (Blaker, 1965b). Gibson (1979) records that in 1932, Carl D. Clarke recommended the standardization of the main light to be from the upper left at 45°. For this reason and because it seems "more natural," we have arranged the main light to be on the left except in those cases when this would throw a shadow in front of the face. Whether light comes from the left or right is less important than that it come from above. Light coming from below appears unnatural because it rarely occurs in nature and thus may cause a reversal in perception of relief, with hills appearing as valleys and vice versa (Blaker, 1977b) (Fig. 3.1). However, the usual "rules" for good lighting include a "main light" to produce modeling and a "fill-in" light to illuminate the shadows to a lower level of intensity.

Types of Lighting

Based on their effect, lighting arrangements have been subdivided into different types and have been classified and described by Gibson (1951) as follows:

1. **Flat Lighting.** This occurs where no shadows are cast in the field of interest, or if there are shadows from one lamp, they are eliminated by illumination from another lamp. Flat lighting is thus subdivided into two types: (a) diffuse and (b) raw. Diffuse lighting is produced, for example, by a single light source in a large reflector covered by a diffuser or by light reflected from a wall or an umbrella. Many flash units mounted on the camera produce this type of lighting if they are over several feet from the subject. Raw flat lighting is produced by two lamps

89

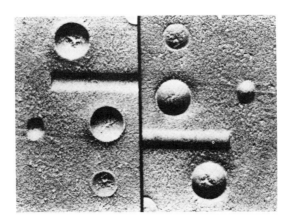

Figure 3.1. Apparent reversal of relief after rotation of the same photograph. Depressions in wet sand were illuminated by a texture light from above and appear as depressions (*left*). When the photograph is rotated 180° (*right*), the depressions appear as elevations. Courtesy of Doctor Charles J. Burton, American Cyanamid Co., and *Journal of Applied Physics.*

of the same intensity with their lighting angles (the angle between the light-subject axis and the lens-subject axis) at 45° (Fig. 3.2). This type of lighting is used for copying and can be used for photographing skin lesions in humans where visibility is due to color and tonal but not textural differences. The 45° lighting angle avoids glare or reflections from flat glistening surfaces but still renders a slight degree of texture.

2. **Axial Lighting.** This occurs when the beam travels along the subject-lens axis and thus the lighting is extremely flat (Fig. 3.3). It is used as supplemental lighting to illuminate the depth of cavities.

3. **Plastic or Modeling Lighting.** This is produced by a "main light" and one or more "fill-in" lights. The main light is used to reveal the morphology of the subject, and the lamp should be moved until the lighting angle that reveals the features of the subject is found. Gibson (1951) states that the observer should mentally ask "Do you notice that fissures . . . ? Can you see the scaly texture . . . ?" Thus, the placement of the main light is critical to reveal the modeling of structures, and shadows should be cast "to bring out the desired details" (Gibson, 1951). We use a lighting angle of 60° with our own standardized equipment (Fig. 3.4).

4. **Texture Lighting.** This is really a modification of modeling lighting where the main light is placed at a low angle to skim across the surface, usually to bring out texture. The lighting angle is usually 75° to 80° (Kodak, 1976) (Fig. 3.5), and as the effect depends on the formation of

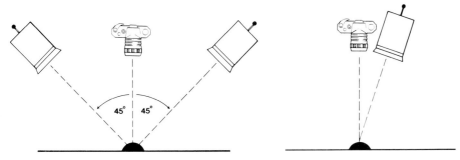

Figure 3.2. Flat lighting from two lamps of equal intensity at 45° lighting angles.

Figure 3.3. Approximately axial lighting.For true axial lighting, the light must travel along the lens's optical axis.

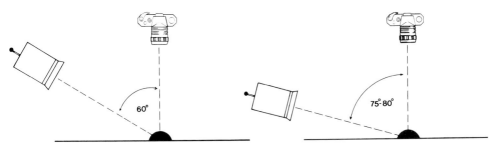

Figure 3.4. Modeling light with the main light at a 60° lighting angle.

Figure 3.5. Texture lighting with the main light at a 75°–80° lighting angle.

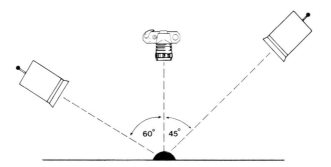

Figure 3.6. Modeling lighting with fill-in illumination at a 45° lighting angle.

sharply defined shadows, a spotlight with a parallel beam of light is more suitable than a diffused light, as for example from a large reflector. In this case, shadow detail is usually of less or of little importance, and fill-in illumination is recommended at the level of ⅙ of that of the main light (Gibson, 1951). This is less fill-in illumination than is normally recommended for use with modeling light. In practice, the skilled photographer can gauge the effect of the fill-in illumination in the viewfinder or by metering the levels of illumination from both the main light and the fill-in lights separately.

5. **Fill-In Illumination.** Once modeling has been achieved by the positioning of the modeling or texture light, the intensity of the shadows usually have to be reduced by fill-in lights. Fill-in illumination should be less intense than that from the modeling lamp, and a 2:1 ratio is usually recommended for color photography and a 4:1 for monochrome photography. These recommendations (Gibson, 1951) were originally made thirty-five years ago when color transparency film had little latitude and could not record detail in both highlights and deep shadows. Many modern transparency films are capable of recording detail in shadows and highlights with a contrast ratio of 3:1. These ratios are determined by taking meter readings at the camera axis, with each light illuminating the subject independently. Fill-in illumination is usually diffused light. If it is close to the subject-lens axis, light may reflect from shiny surfaces. Therefore fill-in illumination for biological materials is frequently at a 45° lighting angle.

There are variations in these recommendations. For scientific photography, Kodak (1970) recommends moving the main light until the significant details are revealed in the image in the viewfinder. However, this recommendation should be done with the reservation that the light come from the top. Shadows are then illuminated with another lamp of one-third of the intensity, aimed directly from above and as close as possible to the camera's optical axis. However, for biological specimens, such axial lighting may result in light being reflected from the specimen into the camera. Therefore, the fill-in lamp is usually placed at 45° (Fig. 3.6). Sometimes, a small accent light, such as a small spot lamp, is used to supply rim lighting or fill-in shadows in deep cavities (Kodak, 1970).

Lighting of Difficult Specimens

Where visibility of a lesion depends on differences in color as, for example, the contrast between the bluish-red consolidated pneumonic areas of a lung and the pale pink normal areas, relatively flat lighting will produce acceptable results. However, when there is little or no difference in color and the lesion is visible because of a change in shape or texture, it may not be visible in a photograph illuminated by flat lighting. A good example is photographing the coning of the cerebellum through the foramen magnum. On the isolated brain, coning is seen as a change in shape and will be most visible when its outline is contrasted with a black background and the specimen is illuminated by modeling lighting.

The best procedure to find the optimal illumination under the standardized lighting system, depicted in Figure 3.7, is to:

1. Turn on the "main" light. This will be either a modeling light at 60° or a texture light at 80° from the lamp's axis to the camera's axis. Compose, frame and focus the camera on the specimen.
2. Manipulate the specimen until the lighting reveals the change in contour desired. This will involve rotating the specimen and its background under the main light and elevating or lowering certain portions of the specimen to obtain the desired viewpoint and illumination.
3. Prop the specimen into the desired position by using modeling clay.
4. Now check the amount of detail visible in the shadows, i.e. lighting contrast. If the shadows are black and devoid of detail so that even the shape of the organ can no longer be seen, add fill-in light from the right lamp which is usually at a 45° lighting angle. In the standard position, this lamp will add as much light as the main light to the specimen, resulting in reduced modeling. This is suitable for specimens with cavities such as an abdominal cavity, but to retain modeling in flatter specimens, the amount of illumination from the fill-in lamp will have to be reduced and this can be done by one of the following methods:
   a. Move the fill-in lamp away from the specimen until the desired degree of fill-in illumination is achieved. This will usually be with the lamp 1-1/2 to 3 times the standard distance from the specimen for color reversal film. Monochrome film, which has a wider latitude and will record shadow detail with more contrasty lighting than color reversal film, will require less fill-in illumination.
   b. If the room is too small so that the fill-in lamp cannot be moved

sufficiently far to reduce its light output, one of the following methods can be used.

(1) On lamps with flood-spot focusing, diffuse the light by moving the focusing lever to "flood."
(2) Rotate the stand so that the shadows are illuminated only by "spill" light from the edge of the lamp.
(3) Turn the lamp so that its light shines on the adjacent *white wall* and bounces onto the specimen.
(4) Add a diffusing screen in front of the lamp to reduce light output. Care must be taken that this is neither flammable nor adds a color cast.
(5) Close the barn doors, or shade portion of the specimen. "Barn doors" are movable metal flaps hinged on the rim of photographic lamps (Fig. 1.4). They can be closed to shade an outer portion of the illuminated field.

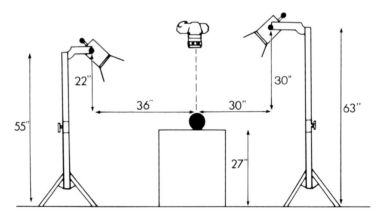

Figure 3.7. Kodak lighting arrangement for color photography of gross specimens. The lighting angles are as in Figure 3.6.

The most desirable options are (1) and (2). If these do not reduce fill-in illumination sufficiently, the only alternative then is to either reduce the amount of light by a diffuser or close the barn doors.

Selecting the correct amount of fill-in illumination takes skill and may have to be learned by experience. The reduction in the intensity of illumination from the fill-in lamp will mean the standardized exposures are no longer valid because the full output of both lamps is not being used. However, this causes little difficulty because the correct exposure will lie between the standard exposure for one and two lamps which is about one stop (Table VII). This range can be easily covered by bracketed exposures.

Standardized Lighting

Standardized lighting using two lamps is commonly used in gross specimen photography, and Vetter (1960) and Currie and Smialowski (1958) point out that even relatively unskilled persons using standardized equipment can obtain good transparencies of the majority of pathological specimens. Color photography of specimens with multiple planes and monochrome photography in general require considerably more expert knowledge and use of complicated lighting and are thus less suited to standardized lighting.

The usual recommendation for lighting arrangements for gross specimens in color photography is to use two lamps at equal distances from the specimen. These distances are measured from the bulb to the subject, not from the lamp stand to the subject. Some authors (Dukes, 1965; Haber, 1980; Vetter, 1984) recommend that both lamps be at 45°, but because this results in flat lighting others prefer the main light at 60° and a fill-in lamp at 45° from the camera axis (Gibson, 1951; Martinsen, 1952; Kodak, 1966; Burgess, 1975). The Kodak arrangement (Fig. 3.7) produces good modeling and, in our experience, works extremely well. When lamps are being placed in a standardized position, the height of the subject has to be assumed. As our average specimen is 3 inches high, the lamp-subject distances were measured from a point 3 inches above the specimen glass (Fig. 3.7). Kodak (1966) emphasizes that precautions must be taken to ensure that raw light from the lamps neither enters the lens directly nor by reflection. Modern macro-lenses usually have built-in lens hoods which extend well beyond the front lens element. Thus, the chances of direct lighting entering the lens are minimal. However reflected light is more difficult to control. Because of the 60° and 45° lighting angles, the Kodak (1966) lamp arrangement (Fig. 3.7) avoids reflections from the specimen glass. However, occasionally, light will be reflected off a shiny background used under the glass. The presence of these reflections should be carefully monitored in the viewfinder. One disadvantage of the Kodak (1966) lighting arrangement is that the light comes from the sides rather than from above the specimen. To minimize this defect, we have moved the main light (at 60°) a few inches towards the top of the frame, the position of the lamp being denoted by an arc on the floor. For black-and-white photographs, the fill-in light is moved to at least 1.5X the distance of the main light from the specimen (Kodak, 1966).

Kodak (1966) recommends two basic positions for the lights: a close one for small specimens and a second with the lamps further away to produce a larger circle of light. Thus, the size of the largest specimen to be photographed is the major controlling factor, and consequently, the first step in calibrating new lights is to check the diameter of the circles of illumination produced by the lights at these recommended distance. Obviously, the closer position has the advantage of higher intensity, thus allowing shorter exposures and should be used if its circle of illumination is sufficiently larger. However, if the lamp stand is too close, its tripod base may impinge on the specimen area. The Kodak (1966) arrangement (Fig. 3.7) produces modeling light with a lighting angle of 60°. For convenience, a texture light with a lighting angle at 80° can be mounted on the same lamp stand beneath the modeling light. Thus, both modeling and texture lights will be available on demand and this greatly speeds photography, as it eliminates the necessity of adjusting the height and the angle of the lamp to obtain texture lighting. Also, errors in positioning the height of the lamp, which would affect exposure in a standardized lighting arrangement, are avoided.

Advantages of Fixed Lamp-Subject Distances
These are:

1. Exposures can be accurately standardized, ensuring a high repeatability of correct exposures even with subjects of different reflectivities and thus reducing the need for bracketing exposures. We bracket only over ½ stop, e.g. f-16–f-19. Many pathological specimens do not lend themselves to accurate metering because they are not the hypothetical "average" subject which reflects 18 percent of the light falling on it and thus the meter is mislead. It is impossible for the majority of camera metering systems to estimate accurately the exposure for subjects such as bleached fixed brain slices on a black background, particularly if the subject/background ratio varies from frame to frame.
2. Exposures can be made very quickly.
3. If additional lighting is required, e.g. a mini-spot to illuminate cavities, in many cases this can be added without altering the standard exposures.

4. The position of the center of the lamp stand is marked as a spot or a small arc on the floor so that the lamp can be moved towards the top of the specimen and yet the lamp-subject distance kept constant.
5. The specimen can be rotated to vary the angle of illumination rather than moving the lights.

Disadvantages of Lights with Fixed Lamp-Subject Distances. The major disadvantage of fixed lighting is that the admonition that "lighting should always be natural and come from above" is partially ignored. In nature, lighting does not come from below, and such lighting appears strange or unnatural ("spook" lighting) and can result in a reversal of perception of relief (Blaker, 1977b) (Fig. 3.1). Many gross specimen photography units not only have fixed lights but also have the camera fixed in the horizontal format. This has the disadvantage that specimens whose anatomic positions dictate that they be placed vertically, are frequently placed horizontally to accommodate the background and camera and thus receive light from both above and below (Figs. 1.4 and 3.7). Unfortunately, this is a common fault, but it can be overcome easily by rotating the camera through 90° on the stand to obtain a vertical format. How to achieve this has been described under "Equipment."

The lack of flexibility of fixed lights can be partially overcome by rotating the specimen and its background. As the background is rotated, the effect of the change of lighting angle on modeling and specular highlights on the specimen can be appreciated in the viewfinder. Also, some organs, e.g. halved kidneys, do not always lie flat and one pole may drop below the line of illumination of a single texture light and thus be in shadow. Tilting the background slightly will expose the whole cut surface to light. Thus, lack of flexibility in the lighting is compensated to some degree by rotating the specimen and its background in relation to the camera, and moving lights on a short arc towards the top of the specimen and yet, at the same time, maintaining standardized distances to insure that exposure times remain constant for the "average" subject (Haeberlein, 1979). Flexibility can be further increased by the use of one lamp to emphasize surfaced modeling and texture. One light may be used with either reduced or no fill-in illumination. The most appropriate lamp to use is the left (main) light at 60° from the camera-subject axis or a "texture" light mounted beneath the main light at 75°–80° from the camera-subject axis. Fortunately, both of these lamps throw a shadow which is outside the field of view of the standard (50mm) lens of a 35mm camera with the passively illuminated light box (Fig. 2.4) for all but the largest specimens. Rarely, the right lamp (45°) alone will provide better illumination for organs with deep cavities (e.g. the opened heart) or give better modeling with less objectionable specular highlights and shadows. Unfortunately, the shadow from this lamp is always visible within the field of view of a 50mm lens, and thus in order to avoid objectionable shadows, the use of the right lamp alone is best confined to those specimens with little or no background.

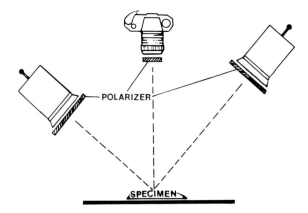

Figure 3.8. Control of specular highlights. Both lights are polarized and specular highlights on specimens are controlled by rotating the polarizer over the camera lens.

Lighting Equipment

In the selection of lights, a major factor to consider is the amount of light delivered to the specimen. This should be sufficient to allow lenses to be used at apertures small enough to obtain adequate depth of field, usually at f-16–f-22, but with exposures short enough to avoid reciprocity failure with either direct or polarized light. Long exposures cause reciprocity failure which results in color shifts and color casts. Also, colors tend to be more saturated the greater the amount of light that falls on them.

Dukes (1975) and Vetter (1984) recommend two 650W tungsten-halogen lamps and one 150W spotlamp. Haeberlein (1979) recommended a main spotlight of 500W to 1000W and a fill-in floodlamp of 500W as well as a 250W mini-spotlight for cavity illumination. Modern spotlights or lamps with focusable filaments to produce either spotlamp- or floodlamp-type lighting have replaced the old variety of lamps with broad reflectors and photoflood bulbs.

Large reflectors fitted with photoflood lamps have the following disadvantages:

1. Inefficient concentration of light and thus the need for longer exposures.
2. Light spilled from reflectors may reflect off walls onto the specimens and cause color casts if the walls are not perfectly white.
3. Cause large specular highlights.
4. Require very large and therefore very expensive polarizing filters.
5. Produce diffuse light which gives poor modeling and texture rendition.
6. Photoflood bulbs used in large reflectors have relatively short lives. More important, due to the deposition of vaporized tungsten on the glass bulb, they tend to darken after half the rated life. This not only reduces light output but also introduces a color cast, usually green. To extend the useful life of photoflood bulbs, rheostats may be used to reduce the light output during focusing and composing of the photograph, and the lamps are run at full voltage only during exposure of the film.

Spotlights. Modern spotlights, particularly the focusable variety, can be adjusted from a hard parallel beam to produce hard shadows and emphasize texture and modeling to a moderately diffuse beam for use as a fill-in light or diffused light for large specimens. Also the reflectors of these spotlights have small diameters, produce small specular highlights and require only small and relatively economical polarizing filters. The light output of a 650W tungsten-halogen bulb in a spotlight reflector allows sufficiently short exposures to avoid reciprocity failure with most modern color films, even with polarizing filters, and the bulbs have long lives. More important, they maintain their color temperature until they burn out. However, if the bulb is touched with bare fingers, the grease from the fingers will burn into the glass and the bulb may break, sometimes explosively. Selection of a spotlight will be a compromise between cost, weight, circle of illumination at the proposed working distance and evenness of illumination as the light is focused from spot to flood (see "Equipment").

Fill-In Lights. Either focusable spotlights (in the "flood" position), lamps in large reflectors or lamps fitted with diffusers all of which produce diffuse lighting, or reflectors made of white cardboard or matte aluminum may be used to supply fill-in illumination. However, Haeberlein (1979) prefers to use a second light source rather than a reflector to lighten shadows, because reflectors cause a "smudging" effect due to large reflections on moist surfaces which leads to falsification of colors and textures. However, reflectors such as sheets of white 8-½ × 11 inch cardboard are very useful as fill-in illumination with glaring white subjects such as formalin-fixed brains. The amount of fill-in light is easily controlled by moving the card towards or away from the specimen, as the effect is judged in the viewfinder.

Lighting When Only Limited Space is Available. In some facilities, only a limited amount of wall or bench space will be available and the standardized lamps, 36 and 30 inches from the subject (Fig. 3.7), will not be able to be accommodated. Kodak (1966) actually has two recommendations for standardized lighting using photofloods: the one depicted in Figure 3.7 for specimens with one dimension greater than 15 inches and the other with lamps only 26 and 21 inches from the subject to produce a circle of illumination 15 inches in diameter. This will accommodate a rectangular frame which will hold a specimen whose longest dimension is 10–11 inches. The total distance from lamp to lamp is 47 inches. If there is insufficient floor space to accommodate lampstands, then wall mounts similar to those in Figure 2.7 can be used. Thus, small specimens can be photographed even if only 4–5 feet of wall space are available. Leapley (1969) described a cabinet for photography of small specimens. This was 60 inches high, 20 inches wide and 32-¼ inches deep. When the doors were opened, two electronic flash units were automatically correctly positioned. Diffusers were used over the flash units to obtain even illumination. Although the cabinet is 20 inches wide with the doors closed, the total width with the doors opened is approximately 80 inches.

The major limitations to this type of photography is the reduction in the flexibility of lighting. Texture lighting and moving lamps to control fill-in illumination are not available. Fill-in illumination can still be regulated by using neutral density filters over the lamp or flash unit or by using flash units whose power output can be reduced to ½, ¼ or ⅛. For the majority of routine small specimens with good color contrast, the photographic results should be good.

Lighting for Laboratory Animal Organs and Cadavers. Because the bodies and organs of laboratory animals are small, they present a problem with depth of field and also require lamps with smaller circles of illumination. Many laboratory animal specimens can be photographed by a camera mounted on a copy stand on the laboratory bench, with the lamps standing on the bench also. Consequently, these lamps need to be smaller than those used for general necropsy room photography. Because organs of laboratory animals are very small, relatively small changes in shape and surface texture need to be accentuated by lighting. For this reason, lamps capable of focusing a parallel beam of light to produce crisp shadows and emphasize small changes in surface texture are necessary, particularly in monochrome photography. Lamps should accept bulbs of the correct color temperature for the film to be used and have slots to accept polarizing filters. Very small specimens can be illuminated by some illuminators designed for use with dissecting microscopes or by integrated units such as the Bogen Light Modulator® (Bogen Photo Corp., Fair Lawn, NJ 07410) which includes a copy stand and top and background lights. This unit has lamps specifically designed to illuminate small fields, and the size of these is controlled by Plexiglas "pipes" which fit into the lamps.

SPECULAR HIGHLIGHTS

The reflections of light sources in a subject are called "specular highlights" or sometimes "catch lights" (Gibson, 1949), and they are an important and common problem in gross specimen photography. The problem of specular highlights has been beautifully described by Beiter et al. (1950), who point out that

> they are usually unnoticed or disregarded when objects are viewed directly, since numerous small movements of the eyes and head made ordinary vision a kind of movie rather than a single view. With a single still picture such compensatory movements cannot be made, so that a highlight, actually no more objectionable than in a single direct view of the original object, now obtrudes.... Whether he is aware of it or not, an observer's attention is likely to be drawn forcibly to the region of a highlight and, if this is not the proper center of interest the meaning of the picture is distorted or lost. The presence of numerous highlights may divide attention to the point where the picture becomes uninteresting or meaningless and, in addition, may obscure many details. For these reasons, considerable effort is often expended, together with much ingenuity, to remove all highlights from a photograph of a gross pathologic specimen.... Unhighlighted objects appear artificial and flat. Few real objects are ever seen without highlights. Highlights enter into our perception of depth and roundness, and, if correctly placed, they may serve the same function in a picture. The aim of our photography, then, should not be the total elimination of highlights,

but their control so that they contribute to the photograph rather than detract from it.

In fact, some delicate transparent membranes can be seen only because of their highlight reflections (Smialowski and Currie, 1960a). Therefore, because of their importance, the factors which control their size and location should be understood so that efforts can be aimed at reduction in size, number and placement.

1. Factors Dependent on Laws of Reflection

Specular highlights are reflections of light sources (Beiter et al., 1950), and consequently their position and size are dependent on the basic law of reflection which states that the angle of incidence equals the angle of reflection. Factors which influence location and size of highlights and are dependent on this law are:

1. Position of lights
   (a) angle between lamp-subject and camera-subject axes, called the lighting angle.
   (b) lamp-subject distance.
2. Size of lights, usually the diameter of the reflector.
3. Position of camera's optical axis in relation to surface of specimen.
4. Specimen orientation.

Even small alterations of any one of the above factors may result in a reduction in highlights. With a fixed camera stand and standardized lights whose lamp-subject distance cannot be changed although the lights can be moved a little on an arc, the only alternatives are to rotate the specimen or tilt the background and evaluate the effect in the viewfinder. When lights are positioned at a very low angle, for example, at 80° from the camera-specimen axis to accentuate texture, few reflections occur from flat surfaces such as slices of brain, liver or kidney, provided that slices are smooth and flat.

The size of the highlights is directly proportional to the diameter of the light source and inversely proportional to the lamp-subject distance. Increasing the number of lights increases the number of highlights. Recommendations are to use lamps with reflectors of small diameter and reduce the number of lights. The lamp-subject distance cannot be used to control specular highlight size easily, because other factors such as the sizes of the circle of illumination at set lamp-subject distances are more important. Older recommendations were to blacken reflectors and use clear bulbs (Beiter, 1946; Kodak, 1966). This reduces the size of the light source to that of the filament. These recommendations are not applicable to focusable spotlamps where the reflector is required to collimate light. However, modern spotlamps have relatively small-diameter reflectors which produce only small specular highlights. With standardized lighting, left and right lights should be tried independently. Often, the use of one light will reduce highlights. If not, the specimen and background can be rotated. Once the optimal position is found, the camera back is rotated to obtain the correct framing of the subject.

Marginal Highlights. Beiter et al. (1950) describe three types of marginal highlights.

1. Reflections of the light source directly from the edge of the specimen. These can be removed by tilting the specimen, by raising or lowering one side of the background or propping up the edge of the specimen with modeling clay. If this fails, Beiter et al. (1950) recommends wetting the edge with saline or kerosene.
2. Reflections of the light source from the top of the glass onto the specimen. These can be blocked by placing thin black blocks of wood or cardboard on top of the glass to prevent reflection of the light. Blocks are moved towards the specimen until the reflections disappear. In our experience, these are more likely to occur with a texture light than with a modeling light.
3. Reflections of the transilluminated background in the top glass. This, like 2, is a reflection of light off the top glass plate, but, in this case, rays originate from underneath and cannot be removed by black cardboard on top of the glass. These reflections have to be blocked by masking off the unused portion of the transilluminated background underneath the top glass.

2. Effect of Specimen Preparation

Flat specimens can be oriented to control specular highlights, but Blaker (1977d) points out that with specimens of irregular shape, altering the position of lights merely serves to move the reflections around. Frequently, reflections come from extraneous fat or loose strands of tissue and blood. Fat and extraneous tissue should be trimmed and the blood dabbed off with lintless soft disposable laboratory paper towels. In our experience, a major source of specular highlights is caused by washing tissues. This is particularly true of serous surfaces and to a lesser extent mucous surfaces. It matters little if the wash is water, physiological saline or Jores' solution. Washing should be avoided and used only as a last resort. Organs and serous surfaces with early postmortem changes also are "edematous" and thus highly glistening and produce numerous specular highlights. Beiter et al. (1950) point out that the number and size of specular highlights may be altered by wetting or drying the specimen. They found that the great majority of fresh specimens had fewer or sharper highlights if the surface was kept wet. This may appear to be contrary to our findings that washing of fresh tissues causes highlights. The key to this discussion is the definition of fresh. Normal organs removed from a recently dead cadaver have few highlights. If organs are washed in water or Jores' solution, the capsule will develop more highlights. If, on the other hand, fresh tissues are allowed to dry out either on the autopsy table or in the refrigerator, the serosa becomes hard and glistening and now reflects light readily to form specular highlights. Thus, each subject should be evaluated on its need. Fresh organs should require no treatment; but if their serosa dries and becomes glistening, its surface should be moistened with physiological saline, as this may reduce specular highlights. It should be emphasized that drying of tissues can take place in minutes under hot, low humidity conditions. Thus, climate control in necropsy and photography rooms is essential (see "Necropsy Photography Room").

Fresh, soft, sagging specimens such as longitudinal sections of unfixed kidneys have curved surfaces which reflect light into the lens no matter how the specimen is rotated or tilted. The curved surface should be made flat by propping up the kidney with modeling clay (Smialowski and Currie, 1960a). An alternative technique for kidneys is discussed next (see 4 below). Because serous surfaces are a major cause of specular highlights, when selecting an organ slice for photography, if possible, choose a face which has no serous surface visible. For example, liver slices have sloping sides covered by serosa. Choosing the larger side obscures the serosal surface. To obtain a completely flat surface, organs such as kidneys should be bisected with a long straight knife using a single stroke. This technique should also be used for slicing brain and liver. Repeated to-and-fro movements cause small ridges on the cut surfaces and these produce numerous specular highlights (Beiter et al., 1950). Knives with blades 12 to 24 inches long are needed as described under "Specimen Preparation."

3. Polarization

The application of polarizing filters to medical photography has been summarized by Haeberlein (1979) who points out that while a single polarizing filter on the camera can eliminate or reduce reflections in sunlight, a single filter on the camera has little effect in artificial light because it is unpolarized. Thus, polarizers are required both on the light to produce polarized light and also on the camera to act as an analyzer to remove reflections (Fig. 3.8). Photographs taken with fully polarized light may appear flat and have reduced definition (Beiter et al., 1950; Haeberlein, 1979), but Haeberlein (1979) has overcome this effect by using two spotlights, one of which is polarized and the other not. The latter is used to produce some localized highlights to make the specimen appear more realistic. Polarization reduces both the intensity and size of highlights even if it cannot completely eliminate them. Polarization may be necessary when other methods fail. Total polarization may be desirable with fixed specimens (Haeberlein, 1979). Polarizers on lamps should not be too close to the bulb, as they may be damaged by the heat (Haeberlein, 1979). Polarizing filters necessitate a considerable increase in exposure, from four to six or even an eight-fold increase (Haeberlein, 1979; Haber, 1980). Thus, lamps should be selected on the basis of their light output which should be sufficient, even after polarization, to allow the use of exposure times short enough to avoid reciprocity failure.

4. Small Specimen Adhered to a Glass Plate

Burry and Stewart (1973) describe a simple but effective method suitable for small unfixed tissues. Cross-sectional slices of kidney (human) were blotted and placed face down on glass (Petri dish). The glass was inverted but the kidney slices remained in position, held by surface tension (Fig. 3.9). Precautions included slicing a perfectly flat slice, ensuring that there were no air bubbles between the glass and specimen, and using a flat uniformly thick glass without imperfections. The technique has also been applied to the photography of slices of liver, spleen, lymph node and brain. The limiting factors are the weight of the tissue that can be supported by surface tension and the ability to obtain a perfectly flat slice. This technique is well worth trying with small specimens. How to obtain uniformly thin sections has been described under "Specimen Preparation." The technique described for cutting brain slices should be tried (Fig. 4.20). In practice, kidney slices frequently have specular highlights reflected from tubules and glomeruli, particularly if these have amyloid deposits, and control of specular highlights is essential to prevent their obscuring important detail.

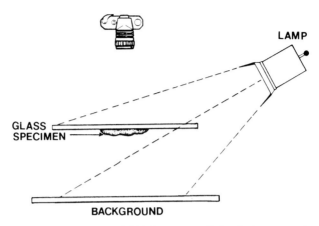

Figure 3.9. Elimination of specular highlights on small fresh tissue specimens. Courtesy of A. F. Burry and B. Stewart and *Medical and Biological Illustration.*

5. Immersion Photography

In this very old technique, the specimen, either an organ or slice of an organ, is completely immersed in a fluid. Tap water, distilled water, physiological saline, alcohol, light mineral oil, xylene, kerosene and glycerine in water have all been used (Martinsen, 1952; Martinsen, 1963). The type of fluid affects the clarity and buoyancy of the specimen (Martinsen, 1963), presumably due to refractive index and specific gravity, respectively. However, physiological saline is recommended with unfixed tissues (Ellis, 1977) and alcohol, if color restoration is being attempted with formalin-fixed tissues (Beiter et al., 1950). Martin (1953) recommends 95 percent alcohol because most specimens sink in it. Immersion has never been popular with the busy photographer (Martinsen, 1952) and pathologists have considerable reservation about the effects of fluid on unfixed tissues. Martin (1953) points out that "except in very expert hands, the finished result often leaves something to be desired; some flattening of contrast is to be expected." This method should be a last resort when all previous ones to control specular highlights have proven to be inadequate. It does have a place in the photography of formalin-fixed specimens, for example, in monochrome photography of the cut surface of the kidney to show amyloid in renal glomeruli or radial bands of fibrous tissue. Without immersion or polarization, these lesions may be obscured by specular highlights.

Immersion is particularly suited to bring out the villous or papillary nature of some tumors (Halsman and Ishak, 1977) or synovial membranes with villous hyperplasia. Also, small tapeworms such as *Echinococcus granulosus* attached to the intestine are revealed beautifully as they float approximately perpendicular to the intestinal mucosa. Good color photographs of fresh specimens are rarely obtained with this technique, since blood oozes from the surface (Beiter et al., 1950). This may not be true of organs such as whole kidneys or strips of intestine if the animal has been exsanguinated at euthanasia.

Preparation of Specimens for Immersion Photography in an Open Tray. The steps are:

1. Wash the organ or tissue in physiological saline (Kodak, 1966) or distilled water (Ellis, 1977). Ellis (1977) found physiological saline causes less cellular swelling than the hypotonic distilled water. Tap water forms excess air bubbles, particularly if the faucet outlet has an aerator.

2. Prepare the tissue. Because of buoyancy, many tissues must be sutured to lead strips to weigh them down (Ellis, 1979), pinned to a board covered by oilcloth (Kodak, 1966), or covered by plate glass or in a special glass-topped tank (Kennedy, 1984) (see below). The first two techniques are not suitable for transillumination.

3. Place the specimen in a flat dish with a flat uniformally thick transparent glass bottom without trade names or indentations. Such dishes are not easy to find, and many commercially available dishes have slightly curved bottoms for increased strength. Del Campo et al. (1974) custom made a dish of $\frac{1}{4}$ inch plate glass glued together by silicone glue. Such dishes can be made by aquarium supply houses. Our's measures $15 \times 15 \times 4$ inches.

4. Barely cover the specimen with immersion fluid. Physiological saline would appear to be the most innocuous for fresh specimens (Ellis, 1977), although Blaker (1977d) recommends distilled water because it has fewer air bubbles. However, air can be driven out of physiological saline by preheating. Alcohol (95%) required for color restoration of formalin-fixed tissues also prevents most tissues from floating. In black-and-white photography of fixed specimens such as heart or muscle to show necrotic of fibrosed areas, color restoration is not necessary. Hansell (1985) indicates that there is a "diffusion swirl, invisible to the naked eye but detrimental to image quality" if tissues are placed in an immersion fluid different from the one they have been submerged in. Therefore, he recommends that specimens should be photographed in the medium

in which they were fixed. This might cause some difficulty with formalin-fixed tissues because of irritant fumes. If the photography room has down-draft airflow (see "Facilities") and not less than 15 air changes per hour, fumes should not be a problem.

5. If the surface of the specimen is not uniformly flat, it can be covered with a piece of flat plate glass (Kodak, 1966). To ensure that no air bubbles are trapped under the glass, one end of it should be lowered first and then the remainder lowered into the solution. Any remaining air bubbles may be removed by tapping (Smialowski and Currie, 1960a). Bubbles on the inside of the jar or on the specimen are removed by a brush or a pointed needle.

Glass-Covered Tanks. Kennedy (1984) overcame the problem of floating specimens and ripples and waves on the surface of the immersion fluid by designing two different glass-covered tanks: one designated a "chimney tank" (Fig. 3.10) for photography of transected eyeballs and a larger one to hold cross sections of heart and lungs (Figs. 3.11 and 3.12). These tanks have a glass window ($1/16$ inch thick) and are filled with fluid to a level higher than the window. The larger one is really a tray with a glass bottom and Plexiglas sides but with two of the sides extending down to support the glass bottom above the specimen in the tank (Fig. 3.11). After the specimen has been placed in the bottom of the tank, the fluid level is raised to the level where the glass of the inner tray would be. Then the tray with its glass bottom is tilted and placed in the tank over the specimen. The mass of the tray raises the fluid level above the level of the glass bottom (Fig. 3.11). This method is quicker than restraining floating specimens with lead weights or waiting for ripples and waves to cease. To reduce air bubble formation, the immersion fluid (physiological saline) for fresh specimens is made from boiled (degassed) water and the inside of the tank and window are coated with a silicone solution (Siliclad®) (Kennedy, 1985). Hansell (1985) criticized the introduction of another refractive medium (glass) between the camera and the specimen, but, because of the absence of surface ripples, results have been excellent (Fig. 3.12).

Lighting for Immersion Photography. Recommendations are to use two lights at 45° (Gibson, 1949; Martinsen, 1952; Kodak, 1966; Ellis, 1977). Usually, incandescent lamps are used, but Brain (1973) used two electronic flash units. Ellis (1977) balanced the transilluminated background against the top lights by using a rheostat. Hansell (1985) recommends the

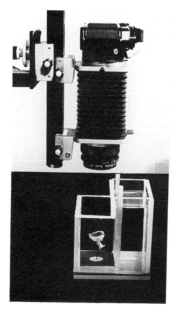

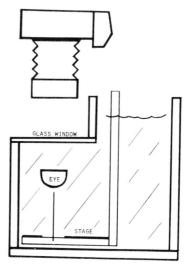

Figure 3.10. "Chimney" tank. This measures approximately 4³/4 inches high, 4¹/2 inches long and 3¹/2 inches wide. The specimen (in this case an eye) is supported on a wire frame attached to a removable Plexiglas background. Courtesy of Mr. L. A. Kennedy and *Journal of Biological Photography.*

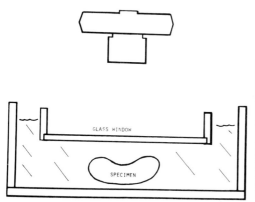

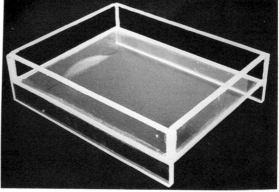

Figure 3.11. Plexiglas tray and "dam lid." (*Left*) Side elevation of dam lid through the middle of the tank. (*Right*) The window in the bottom of the tray is supported by two Plexiglas side plates. The outer tray measures approximately 10 × 8 × 1 inches. Courtesy of Mr. L. A. Kennedy and *Journal of Biological Photography.*

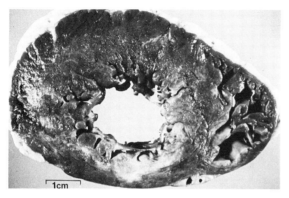 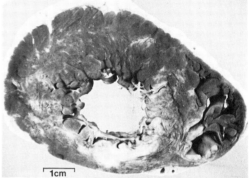

Figure 3.12. Cross section of both ventricles of a heart with myocardial fibrosis following myocardial infarction. The specimen is stained for succinic dehydrogenase with tetrazolium blue. Areas of fibrosis are pale. (*Right*) Note that in the immersed specimen the pale fibrotic areas are readily seen. (*Left*) In an unimmersed specimen, specular highlights obscure some of these areas and are distracting. Courtesy of L. A. Kennedy and *Journal of Biological Photography.*

use of submersible flexible fiber-optic light guides. These would allow more control of illumination than the flat even lighting from two lamps at 45°.

Backgrounds for Immersion Photography. Either a transilluminated background (light box), black box or black velvet can be used. Villous hyperplasia of synovial membranes of joints is best depicted with a black background to emphasize the outline of the villi. The factors involved in selecting backgrounds are discussed under "Backgrounds."

Equipment Required. If the Kennedy tanks are not used, this includes:

- metric rulers
- lead strips
- black suture materials and needles
- ⅝ inch diameter clear Plexiglas rod to elevate ruler
- lead to weigh ruler down
- transilluminated background and black box
- immersion tank or large Petri dish for small specimens
- immersion fluid, physiological saline, 95% alcohol or 10% NBF

Disadvantages of Immersion Photography in an Open Tray. Because shadows are cast by the top edges of the sides, the tank needs to be large enough to avoid these shadows being cast on the specimen (Haeberlein, 1979). Unfortunately, this requires a large container which is heavy, difficult to move (Haeberlein, 1979) and in which fluid stays in motion

for many minutes. Brain (1973) recommends that the sides of the recepta-
cle be white and opaque (e.g. white opaque Perspex®) to reflect light onto
the subject. Buoyant specimens have to be weighed or pinned down
(Ellis, 1977). This is particularly true of air or gas-filled organs such as
lungs and intestine (Schmidt and Haulenbeck, 1932). Immersion fluids
(e.g. distilled water) may damage the specimen histologically (Haeberlein,
1979; Ellis, 1977) or modify color (Haeberlein, 1979). Jores' fluid, for
example, enhances red colors. Fluids easily become turbid from blood or
exudate, especially if the fluid or specimen is moved. To maintain a clear
colorless solution, Smialowski and Currie (1960a) designed a tank with a
continuous exchange of fluid (Fig. 3.13). However, immersion photography of fresh specimens with its problem of blood staining the immersion
fluid is extremely time consuming. Underfluid artifacts such as air-
bubbles may be present in and around the tissue (Ellis, 1977). Water and
air bubbles may be present between the bottom of the glass tank and the
glass of the light box. Immersion photography involves delay; it is
necessary for all fluid movement to stop so that the papillary and the
villous surfaces stop swaying in the fluid. The final apearance is frequently disappointing. Without highlights, the tissue appears "dead."
There is a reduction in color saturation and contrast and a lack of round-
ness and modeling because superficial crevices and depressions are filled
with water (Opps, 1934). Nevertheless, like polarized light photography,
immersion photography has a place in the photography of fixed specimens
(Haeberlein, 1979). Investment in the Kennedy tanks would be well worth
it for any laboratory doing much of this type of photography.

Summary

Specular highlights are a problem in gross specimen photography but
can be reduced with a fixed lighting arrangement by the following
techniques:

Specimen Preparation

1. Fresh specimens. Have minimum delay between death and photography to reduce autolysis which can cause "edema."
2. Avoid rinsing specimens, particularly serosa and mucosa in any
   fluid.
3. Cut slices with absolutely flat surfaces by using knives sufficiently
   long to cut the organ in one slice without a sawing motion which
   produces a serrated surface.

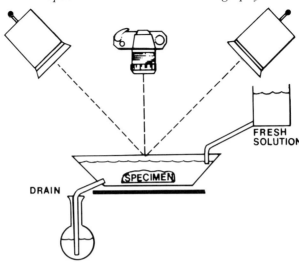

Figure 3.13. Immersion photography. Method of exchanging fluid. Redrawn with permission of authors. From Smialowski, A. and Curry, D. J., 1960, *Photography in Medicine.*

4. Remove all tags of tissue, fat, blood, etc.
5. Prop curved surfaces, e.g. cut surface of fresh kidney into a flat plane with modeling clay.
6. Adhere small specimens to the underside of a glass plate.
7. If the above methods fail, try blotting or adding moisture to the surface of tissue slices. Check the effect in the viewfinder.

Optical Considerations

1. Use the minimum number of lights.
2. Use small reflectors.
3. Compare the effect of left and right lights alone.
4. Rotate and tilt specimen or background to change the angle of incidence of light.

Polarized Light. If all of the above techniques fail, polarize one or both lights to produce polarized light and add an analyzer to the camera lens. Photographs of formalin-fixed tissue may be improved by polarized light.

Immersion Photography. This is really only applicable to fixed specimens when no polarizers are available or if polarization fails to remove sufficiently the highlights. Immersion photography should be used for those specimens such as fixed myocardium, muscle, transected eyes and kidneys where specular highlights significantly obscure detail. Immersion photography is particularly applicable to papillary and villous surfaces even in fresh specimens if oozing of blood is absent.

ORIENTATION OF SPECIMENS

Despite the obvious necessity of photographing specimens in their correct anatomical positions and the exhortations of several authors (Vetter, 1960; Kodak, 1970; Burgess, 1975), there is little sympathy for this requirement, and incorrectly oriented specimens are common in books and journals on human pathology and even more common in those on veterinary pathology. Viewing of some photographs becomes an exercise in solving the puzzle as to which side should be up. Martin (1961) states that it is desirable that the "finished picture depict the subject in, as near as possible, its true anatomic relationship and, additionally, the right way up," as it is "manifestly absurd to produce the picture upside down." Thus, Vetter (1960) points out that organs are placed in a position as would be seen by a viewer facing the (human) patient. There are exceptions. Brain slices are always placed so that their caudal surfaces are viewed and thus the left side of the brain slice is always on the viewer's left. This allows the viewer to orient himself easily and reliably, making correlation of lesions with clinical findings easier.

While there is relatively little doubt about the correct orientation of human and thus primate organs, some confusion exists over the correct orientation of organs of quadrupeds. A good basic rule is that if the ventral or dorsal surfaces of organs are to be photographed, organs should be placed in the position they would occupy when the axis of the body is vertical and the animal is in ventral or dorsal recumbency. The convention is to put the head to the top of the frame. If organs of quadrupeds are placed in the position they occupy while the animal is standing erect, the views would be of the *lateral* surfaces of those organs. The common mistake is to view the dorsal or ventral surfaces of organs such as the urinary and female reproductive tracts and lungs in a horizontal format (Fig. 3.14). This results in one kidney or ovary or uterine horn being above the other which is anatomically incorrect. Thus, the logical procedure when dorsal or ventral surfaces of organs of quadrupeds are to be photographed is to arrange them as is done for humans with the cranial pole towards to the top of the frame and with their longitudinal axes vertical (Fig. 3.15). However, photographs of the lateral surfaces of organs such as lungs should be positioned as in the erect animal viewed from the side and thus in a horizontal format (Fig. 3.16).

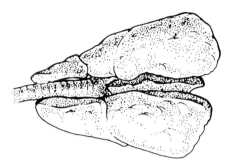

Figure 3.14. Quadruped lungs in incorrect anatomic position. This position is usually selected to suit a horizontal camera format.

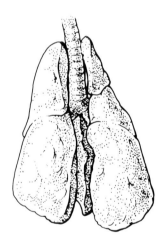

Figure 3.15. Correct anatomic position for dorsal and ventral views of lungs of all animals. The cranial poles are at the top of the frame. This dictates the use of a vertical camera format.

The importance of correct orientation is best shown in testes of domestic animals, discussed in detail under "Specimen Preparation." The long axes of the testes of different species are not oriented in the same direction. In carnivores they are horizontal and in ruminants vertical. Thus, photographs of correctly oriented testes are educational, illustrating differences between species.

Thus, in summary, the convention applied to positioning organs is

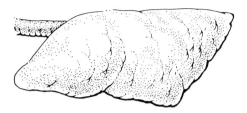

Figure 3.16. Lateral surface of quadruped lung in correct anatomic orientation. For this, a horizontal camera format is required.

that either the cranial "end" of organs such as the kidney and uterus or dorsal borders of organs such as the liver, heart, testis and brain slices should always be positioned towards the top of the photographic frame. If organs such as the brain and liver are viewed from their caudal surfaces, their left side will be on the left of the photographic frame. However, if the ventral surface of organs such as the kidneys and ovaries are viewed, the kidneys will be reversed.

One reason for the frequency of incorrect orientation is the inability of the photographer to change the framing of a 35mm camera from a horizontal to a vertical format. In fact, most copy or photographic stands make no provision for this change; an exception is the Bogen Maxi Repro Stand. A device to change from horizontal to vertical format easily is now marketed under the name of Vertaflip® (The Saunders Group, 67 Deep Rock Rd., Rochester, NY 14624-3598). It was originally designed to hold a small flash unit to the side of a camera and allows the flash to swivel so that it remains at the top of the frame when the camera is turned to obtain a vertical format. When the Vertaflip is used on a copy stand, there is some vibration and the device is best used with electronic flash lighting.

Many light boxes are rectangular and this also unconsciously biases the photographer to place a long specimen such as a long bone in a horizontal format, even though its correct anatomic position is vertical. It could be argued that specimens in a horizontal format lighted by one lamp on to the top of the specimen could be rotated later during projection. This is true, but it is easy for the photographer to use two lamps and then when the slide is projected in a vertical format, illumination appears to come from above and below. This is unnatural lighting. Also, if the ruler is photographed at the bottom of the frame, it will be out of position on the side after the slide is rotated. The safest arrangement is to use a square background, place the specimen in its anatomic position with the ruler at the bottom and then illuminate it with light from the top or towards the top so that shadows are cast downwards.

COMPOSITION

Good composition means that the viewer's attention is automatically directed towards those portions of the subject that the photographer wants to emphasize. Gross specimen photography gives relatively little freedom to the photographer to control composition, but factors which the photographer can influence are:

1. Distractions such as tissue or props that lead the eye away from the subject towards the background or out of the picture.
2. Framing and proportioning. The latter is the ratio of the area of the specimen to the area of the background, i.e. the percentage of the frame covered by the specimen.
3. Selection of backgrounds which will direct attention either to the border of the specimen or into the specimen.
4. Third's rule.

1. Distractions

Inclusion of several tissues, particularly from the same organ in the one frame, is a common cause of distraction. Halsman and Ishak (1977) recommend that only one coronal section of brain through a lesion be included, because "all the sections of the brain arranged like sausages on a tray makes each individual section proportionately smaller, and it confuses and probably irritates the viewer." For the same reason, multiple liver and lung slices are not recommended. Inclusion of more than one slice is justified only if the intent is to show the *extent* of the lesion throughout the organ. Both halves of a bisected kidney can be included if the photograph is designed to show both external and internal surfaces. Pointers, probes, retractors and labels are clutter and are contraindicated in gross specimen photographs. They have been discussed individually under "Backgrounds."

2. Framing

The usual admonition is to "fill the frame," but this can be overdone. The old portrait adage that the "head should have room to breath" also applies to specimen photography. It is better to have a little excess space around a specimen than to have it too tightly framed (Fig. 3.17). The penalty for framing too closely is that the specimen may touch the edge of the frame and lead the eye out of the picture. Also, problems arise when slides are duplicated. Duplication usually results in a slight increase in magnification, and while there may have been adequate clearance between the specimen and the edge of the frame in the original slide, the specimen may be close to or touch the edge in the duplicate.

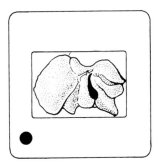 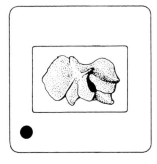 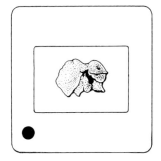

Figure 3.17. (*Left*) Subject touches the borders of the frame. This is undesirable, as it leads the eye out of the frame. (*Center*) Subject fills the frame but is still surrounded by an adequate margin which isolates it visually. (*Right*) Subject is too small and does not fill frame.

In negatives, framing is less critical because the final cropping can be done on the print. Anon (1942) and Kodak (1966) recommended photographing human specimens at fixed ratios of reproduction of 1:1, 1:2, 1:5, and 1:10. However, this policy has the severe disadvantage that often the whole of the frame is not utilized, and also, such an approach is unnecessary if a scale is inserted. If fixed ratios of reproduction are used, the photographer loses control over proportioning and thus the specimen/background ratio may not be optimal to direct the viewer's attention. Fixed RR's are more appropriate to photography of human dermatologic lesions rather than in veterinary pathology and biology where sizes of animals vary enormously.

3. Selection of Background

Inappropriate backgrounds can divert attention, e.g. black backgrounds can rivet the attention of the viewer on the specimen-background margin, even though the major lesion may not be at the border but in the middle of the specimen. A full review of the effect of backgrounds has been given under "Backgrounds."

4. Third's Rule

Kodak (1971) described the "third's rule." The "strong" points of any composition are at the junction of thirds, and normally the points of interest would be placed at or near these (Fig. 3.18). Occasionally, this can be done with gross pathological specimens. However, with most gross lesions the usual suggestion is to put the "focal point in the center of the field and fill the frame" (Halsman and Ishak, 1977). However, the photographer should attempt to produce a visually pleasing composition. Because correct orientation of a specimen is fixed, the only variable to control composition is the area of the specimen included in the frame, if this is not an isolated organ. Thus, composition depends on the balance between the following factors:

1. filling the frame with the area of interest of the specimen.
2. including sufficient of the surrounding tissues to allow the viewer to orient himself.
3. positioning the center of interest to maintain anatomic orientation and yet, if possible, leading the viewer's eye through the important structures of the specimen.

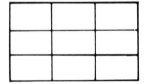

Figure 3.18. Third's Rule. The "strong" points of composition are at the junctions of third's.

In practice, this is done by raising and lowering the camera on the vertical photographic stand, refocusing, and repositioning the specimen by moving the background until the most aesthetically pleasing but informative arrangement is obtained. Occasionally, an arrangement of the specimen will result in a photograph in which many viewers do not see the point of interest. In one of our slides, a large thrombo-embolus in a pulmonary artery in the lung was not detected by many viewers. The field included heart and some lung, but the combination of position of the thrombus and the absence of highlights on it resulted in the eye not being attracted to the main subject. Therefore, if in doubt, several compositions should be taken including "placing the specimen in the center of the field," which is usually considered the least aesthetically desirable position.

FOCUSING AND DEPTH OF FIELD

Focusing

Focusing of most modern single-lens-reflex camera is relatively simple, as the image is bright because the lens aperture automatically opens to its widest opening. A major requirement for specimen photography is to select a focusing screen on which focusing can take place over the whole area. Some focusing screens have circles, stigmometer rangefinders, central microprism and collars and areas on which focusing does not take place. None of these specialized focusing screens are suitable for close-up specimen photography. Therefore, when selecting equipment, it is essential to choose either a camera which accepts interchangeable focusing screens or one whose built-in screen provides focusing anywhere on the screen (full-frame focusing). The only other alternative is to have a full-frame focusing screen installed by a camera repairman. We use a Nikon E screen (Fig. 1.10) which not only allows focusing over its whole surface but also has a pattern of vertical and horizontal lines which facilitates alignment of specimens such as a vertical row of brain slices (Fig. 4.21). A full-frame focusable screen is essential for specimen photography, because the point of interest and therefore the area which should be brought into sharpest focus may be anywhere in the field of view.

The ratio of reproduction (RR) is defined as the ratio between the linear size of an image on the film plane to the linear size of the real object. Thus, at RR = 1 the image on the film plane is life-size. Once the size of the film frame is known, then the size of the specimen field can be calculated easily. For example, the film frame size of a 35mm camera is 36mm × 24mm (approximately 1-½ × 1 inches); therefore, at RR = 1:4, the image is a ¼ normal size and the field of view is 6 inches × 4 inches. Many lenses have RR's calibrated on their barrels. Alternately, the RR's can be quickly determined reasonably accurately by measuring the length of a ruler in focus across the width of the 35mm film frame. As its width is almost 1 inch, if 4 inches of ruler are visible then the RR = 1:4 approximately. The accuracy of this method depends on the accuracy of the viewfinder, since the field of view visible in the viewfinder may be smaller than the image on the negative. Determination of RR is important if one wishes to use it to calculate exposure corrections for the so-called "close-up factors" (Table IX) or to check the depth of field at different apertures (Table IV).

Table IV
EFFECT OF APERTURE ON DEPTH OF FIELD AT RR'S 1:10–1:1

RR	Field Size of 35mm Camera in Inches	Depth of Field in mm		
		f-11	f-16	f-22
1:10	15 × 10	81	117	162
1:8	12 × 8	53	77	106
1:6	9 × 6	31	45	62
1:4	6 × 4	15	21	30
1:3	4½ × 3	9	13	18
1:2	3 × 1½	4.4	6.4	8.8
1:1	1½ × 1	1.5	2.1	3

SOURCE: Morgan and Lester (1956).

Depth of Field

It is critical that the reader have an understanding of what is meant by "depth of field." A full review of the optical factors involved is beyond the scope of this chapter, but its practical significance is extremely important. Although only one plane of the specimen is perfectly in focus on a film plane, there is a distance, both in front of and behind the plane in focus, where the image is brought into "acceptable" focus on the film plane. This acceptable focus is based on the diameter of the so-called "circle of confusion" and the resolution of the human eye. Resolution is defined as the ability of the lens or film to separate two points or lines and mathematically, resolution $= \frac{1}{2}f$ where f is the aperture.

Table IV illustrates that depth of field, which is dependent on two factors—RR and lens aperture (f), decreases as the RR approaches 1:1 and increases as the camera aperture becomes smaller, i.e. the f-number becomes larger. Increasing the depth of field by closing the lens diaphragm (i.e. reducing the diameter of the aperture) has penalties, and Table V illustrates that as the lens aperture is closed, the *theoretical* resolution of the lens becomes less. Thus, a compromise has to be made between theoretical resolution and depth of field of a lens. Few lenses attain their theoretical resolution at apertures approaching full aperture, and most lenses do not give their maximum resolution until they have been stopped down approximately 2–2-½ stops, e.g. from a maximum aperture of f-3.5 to f-8. Kodak (1978) demonstrated that the definition of highly corrected apochromatic process lenses (lenses used in preparing copy for printing) was improved by stopping down from full aperture (f-11 on these lenses) to f-16 or f-22. However, further stopping down reduced sharpness and resolution (Table V).

Table V
EFFECT OF APERTURE ON RESOLUTION OF A THEORETICALLY PERFECT LENS
FOR GREEN LIGHT

	Aperture (f-number)									
	2	*2.8*	*4*	*5.6*	*8*	*11*	*16*	*22*	*32*	*64*
Resolution lines/mm	1000	714	500	357	250	181	125	90	62	31

SOURCE: Gibson (1952) and Mutter (1957).

Another determining factor is the resolving power of the film used. If the resolving power of the lens exceeds that of the film, the limiting factor to resolution is the resolving power of the film. Thus, the aperture of a lens can be closed down to an aperture whose theoretical resolving power almost equals that of the film without affecting the resolution of the image on the film itself. This is not absolutely true, as Mutter (1957) found that resolution of a fast film was 35 lines/mm with a lens resolving 100 lines/mm, but the same film resolved 40–50 lines/mm when used with a lens resolving 300 lines/mm. Table VI illustrates the resolving ability of Kodak color films. Reference to Tables V and VI shows that for Kodachrome 40, the aperture could be reduced to f-19 to match the resolution of the lens with that of the film. The objective is to obtain maximum depth of field without reducing the resolution of the lens below that of the film, and for this reason apertures between f-11 and f-22 are often recommended for close-up photography. These are "effective" apertures, not "relative" apertures (see "Lens Apertures" under "Exposure"). The aperture can be reduced to f-22 if the depth of field is extremely shallow, as there is little point in having acceptable resolution if the image is out of focus. Gibson (1952) recommended f-16 and f-22 as the apertures for maximum resolution with good depth of field for monochromatic and color films, respectively. These recommendations applied to 1952 films. As modern color films have higher resolution, a slightly wider aperture (f-19 or f-16) is recommended for Kodachrome 40 so that its resolution is not reduced.

Exactly how shallow depth of field is in close-up photography can be

Table VI

RESOLUTION AND GRAININESS OF KODAK COLOR TRANSPARENCY FILMS

Film	Resolution	Graininess
Kodachrome 40	100 lines/mm	extremely fine
Kodachrome 25	100 lines/mm	extremely fine
Kodachrome 64	100 lines/mm	very fine
Ektachrome 200	125 lines/mm	very fine

SOURCE: Hurtgen (1978).

appreciated by referring to Table IV. Obviously, for images greater than RR = 1:6 the depth of field of 45mm at *f*-16 will be adequate for many specimens, but as the RR approaches one, depth of field rapidly becomes shallow and is only 2.1mm at RR = 1:1 at *f*-16. Thus, the selection of the aperture is a compromise between resolution and depth of field. To make maximum use of the depth of field when this is extremely narrow, the specimen may have to be reoriented so that the plane of principal focus passes through important structures. Focusing is done at full aperture. Usually, the depth of field extends ⅓ in front (i.e. towards the camera) of the plane of principal focus and ⅔ behind it. However, in close-up photography as RR = 1:1 is approached, the depth of field is almost equal in front of and behind the principal plane of focus (Kodak, 1972b). This fact must be taken into account when focusing specimens. However, if the depth of field is inadequate to allow the whole specimen to be in focus, there are three alternatives. One is to focus so that the important structures are sharply focused and accept that the rest will be out of focus. Kodak (1977b) recommends that "it is better to favor the near detail; slight out-of-focus blurs are more distracting in front of the subject than behind it." The second alternative is to select a smaller RR whose depth of field is adequate to cover the specimen. This will mean that the subject may not fill the frame. The RR necessary to have adequate depth of field can be selected by referring to Table IV. Williams (1984) has described a third alternative: increasing the depth of field by immersing the subject in a fluid whose refractive index is higher than that of air. He states that "since the depth of field is dependent upon the refractive index of the medium between the subject and the camera, increasing the refractive index decreases the apparent depth of the subject thereby increasing the actual depth of field." Water with a refractive index of 1.33 can be used. Immersion photography is accompanied by all of the disadvantages described above.

It is important to realize that the method of focusing is a little different as the RR approaches 1:1. If focusing is done in a conventional manner by turning the focusing mount of the lens, the lens-film plane distance is changed and this changes the magnification or RR. Thus, the easy way to focus is to select the appropriate RR and then move the camera as a whole. With a vertically mounted camera, this is easily done by moving the camera down while simultaneously focusing the camera until the desired magnification (RR) and framing are selected. However, if a subject is to be focused at say RR = 1:2 (half life-size, a field size of 2 × 3 inches with a 35mm camera), the easiest method is to set the lens focusing mechanism to RR = 1:2, or a little less, and focus the camera by lowering it. The final fine focusing can be carried out by moving the camera's lens mount. Thus, the whole procedure can be done very rapidly on a vertically mounted camera with a so-called macro-lens.

EXPOSURE

Many modern cameras have either automatic exposure devices or exposure meters which allow selection of the "correct exposure" by centering a needle. Unfortunately, these devices do not always work correctly with pathological specimens. This is not because the meters are defective but because the subjects are not "average." All exposure meters are calibrated on the assumption that the subject is "average" and reflects 18 percent of the light falling upon it. This is the reflectance of the Kodak Neutral Test Card. However, caucasian skin reflects approximately 36 percent of the light falling on it, and subjects such as slices of fixed brain reflect even more. The problem of metering the correct exposure for pathological specimens is compounded when the camera also meters the background, which with pathological specimens can vary from white to grey to black. Obviously, an exposure meter reading a subject such as a white fixed brain slice on a black background will be markedly influenced by the percentage of the field occupied by each. Thus, the meter will indicate a different exposure for a brain slice surrounded by a black background as compared to a field completely covered by the same brain slice. The correct exposure would remain constant if the light falling on the specimen is fixed in intensity.

The effect of the reflectance of the specimen and background and the proportion of each viewed by the camera, e.g. white brain slices on a black background which so badly mislead exposure meters reading *reflected* light, can be overcome by using an incident light meter which reads the light *falling* on the specimen. Another alternative is to use a reflected light meter reading a Kodak Neutral Test Card (18% reflectance). These techniques work well for ordinary photography, but, because the distance between the camera and the specimen is small in specimen photography, it is difficult to maneuver the meter and card without either casting a shadow on the card or contaminating the card by touching it on the specimen. The card can be metered with the camera's through-the-lens metering system, but, in our experience, results are not always reliable, particularly when texture light (80° from the camera's axis) is used. Also, the method is slower, less convenient and less reliable than using standardized exposures.

Exposure Standardization

This is based on standardized lighting (see "Lighting") and is the basis of our solution to this problem. This method has been described by Smialowski and Currie (1950) and Vetter (1960). By a series of trials, the correct exposure for a subject on a color transparency film is determined. One easy way to do this is to photograph caucasian skin such as a hand or fingers. The hand can be metered and the correct exposure should be approximately twice the exposure indicated on the exposure meter for the hand alone. In other words, the meter needs to be close enough to the subject so that its angle of acceptance is completely filled by the subject alone, and thus the meter "sees" no background. Once the correct exposure for caucasian skin has been confirmed by exposing a test role of film, the next step is to determine the correct exposures for a variety of subjects such as thoracic and abdominal viscera, light subjects such as fixed brain slices and dark subjects such as liver, spleen and dark skin. How much exposure correction is needed for light or dark tissues will depend on the latitude and contrast of the film and will vary from one type of color film to another. These corrections can be determined by bracketing exposures above and below the exposure for skin, by 2 stops at ½-stop intervals. The average photographer has little difficulty in evaluating a correctly exposed transparency. The usual advice is to expose for the highlights, which means that these bright areas should not be overexposed even if there is inadequate detail in the shadows. However, the standardized lighting is relatively low in contrast and problems with excessive contrast will usually be due to the subject itself, such as black and white haired skin. The correct exposure for the white hair will result in underexposure of the black; correct exposure of the black will result in overexposure of the white. In such a case, the compromise would be to give the maximum exposure which will not overexpose the white hair and accept that the black will be underexposed.

For reasons discussed under "Close-up Exposure Factors," it is *critical* that the RR used for these trials be kept absolutely constant. If a human hand is photographed at RR = 1:4 (field size of 6 × 4 inches with a 35mm camera), the hand will completely fill the frame and the effect of background on the exposure meter will be eliminated. A table of exposures can be made for the standardized lighting. However, the exposures will be made at an RR = 1:4 and will thus include the close-up exposure factor for this RR, which is 1.5X (Table IX). Therefore, to establish standardized exposures for larger fields where there is no exposure correction, this exposure will have to be increased by a factor of 1.5. Thus, if the correct exposure was determined to be 1/8 second at f-11 at RR = 1:4 with a lens that did not have an automatically compensating diaphragm, the basic exposure for an RR where no correction for close-up exposure factors is required would be 1/8 second at f-13.

Table VII lists the exposures for average gross specimens illuminated by either one or two 650W lamps with the Kodak standardized lighting arrangement and using Kodachrome 40. For dark subjects such as liver, the aperture is opened 1/2 to 1 stop and for black subjects such as the black skin of an Angus cow the aperture is opened 1-1/2 stops. A full "stop" is the interval between the marked apertures on the camera lens (e.g. from f-8 to f-11). Opening the lens one full stop allows twice the amount of light to pass. For fine control of the exposure, the lens can be opened by half a stop. Half stops are usually marked by a dot and not by numbers as on most lenses. The usual apertures marked are the full stops which are f-2, 2.8, 4, 5.6, 8, 11, 16, 22, and 32. The mathematical values of intermediate 1/2 stops and 1/3 stops are given in Table VIII. However, some modern meters with digital readouts will not use these numbers but will give the value between full stops as a decimal (e.g. f-11.5). This number indicates the half stop between f-11 and f-16 which is mathematically 13.4. Similarly, f-11.3 designates the third stop between f-11 and f-16 which mathematically is correctly f-14. Thus, the digital readout is easy to follow although not strictly mathematically correct.

Select the correct exposure from a table (e.g. Table X). For a specific film, the following factors have to be considered:

Table VII
SPECIMEN PHOTOGRAPHY
STANDARDIZED EXPOSURES FOR KODACHROME 40
FOR NIKON MICRO–NIKKOR LENS
WITH AUTOMATICALLY COMPENSATING DIAPHRAGM
AVERAGE SUBJECT

Shutter Speed	*2 Lamps**	*1 Lamp*
⅛ *sec*	f-19	f-13.5

Light subject such as whole fixed brain.............................close ½ stop.
Very light subject such as slices of formalin-fixed bleached brain...........close 1 stop.
Dark subject such as liver ....open ½ stop.
Black subject such as Angus hide ....open 1 stop.

*Colortran Multi-6 lamps with 650W bulbs, 42 inches from the subject.

1. Number of lights
2. Reflectivity of the specimen
3. Close-up exposure factors

Shutter Speed

To minimize variables, the shutter speed for gross specimen photography can be kept constant. Any shutter speed between ⅛ second and 1/500 second is suitable to avoid reciprocity failure. However, the actual shutter speed to give correct exposure will depend on the aperture selected. In other words, the aperture, usually between f-11 and f-22, is selected first to obtain adequate depth of field. Then, the appropriate shutter speed to give the correct exposure is chosen. Fast shutter speeds have the advantage of minimizing vibrations, but these are better eliminated in the design of the equipment. However, very slow shutter speeds may induce "reciprocity failure." The slow shutter speed at which this effect first occurs is usually listed in the manufacturer's literature. Most Kodak professional films do not have reciprocity failure between 1/10 and 1/1000 second exposure (Kodak, 1983). Exposure is controlled by a combination of shutter speed and lens aperture and the same amount of light can be transmitted by a fast shutter speed and a wide lens aperture (e.g. 1/500 second at f-2) or a slow shutter speed with a small lens aperture (e.g. ⅛ second at f-16). Although the same amount of light reaches the film from these two combinations of shutter speeds and lens apertures (Fig. 1.11), the responses of the film may differ. With black-and-white film, reciprocity failure results in additional exposure being required to

Table VIII
NUMERICAL DESIGNATION OF FULL, HALF AND THIRD STOPS BETWEEN *f*-2.8 and *f*-22

Full Stops	2.8			4			5.6			8			11			16			22
Half Stops			3.4			4.8			6.7			9.6			13.4			19		
Third Stops		3.2		3.5		4.5		5		6.3		7		9		10		12.5	14	18	20

Opening the aperture increases light transmission by $2\times$ for a full stop, by $1.4\times$ for half stop and by $1.25\times$ for $1/3$ and $2/3$ stops, respectively.

produce the same density on the film at shutter speeds longer than $^1\!/_{10}$ second. This is not a difficult problem to overcome, and manufacturers provide tables indicating the increase in exposure required.

However, the situation with color films is more difficult. Not only is additional exposure required but, because the three layers of the color film fail at different rates, color casts are produced. These can be removed by using color compensating filters over the lens, but as these absorb some light exposure is further increased by what are designated "filter factors." It is wiser to select a shutter speed in the range for which there is no reciprocity failure. The combination of intensity of illumination and sensitivity (speed, ISO rating) of the film should allow selection of an aperture which allows the optimal compromise between depth of field and resolution (see "Focusing and Depth of Fields"). Thus, the original selection of lamps and film will determine if reciprocity failure will be a problem with exposures using small apertures in the range of f-16 to f-22.

Lens Apertures

These are indicated by numbers engraved on the lens mount and are a source of confusion to many. While a knowledge of their effect on exposure, resolution and depth of field is not critical in "ordinary" photography, it is necessary in "close-up" (RR's 1:20–1:2) and macro-photography (RR's 1:2–30:1) for a basic understanding of their role. The aperture of the lens (f number) is a mathematical ratio expressing the light-transmitting ability of the lens. A lens is usually fitted with an iris diaphragm to close down, or "stop" down the lens aperture, to control the amount of light transmitted. The widest opening of this iris diaphragm is called the *maximum aperture* and is engraved on the lens mount (e.g. f = 1:2, 50mm, etc.). Note that the engraving really states that f = 1:2 or f = 1:2.8, but the common photographic parlance is to call these numbers f-2 or f-2.8. The f-number is defined as diameter of lens in millimeters divided by focal length in millimeters. Thus, in the above example, for a 50mm f-2 lens, the formula is really

$$f = 1:2 = \frac{\text{diameter of lens in mm}}{\text{50mm}} = 25\text{mm}$$

Thus the maximum diameter of the lens or iris is 25mm. Actually, it is slightly more complicated than this. The front lens element may have a greater diameter to prevent vignetting or other optical defects. As the lens is stopped down, the lens aperture becomes smaller and for a 50mm lens at f-16, the diaphragm would have a diameter of:

$$f = 1:16 = \frac{X}{50} = 3mm$$

Thus, closing down the lens and selecting a larger f-number reduces the light transmission through the lens. The f-number in the series is the preceding number multiplied by the square root of 2. This gives the series f-2, f-2.8, f-4, etc. (Table VIII). The significance of the one-stop interval is that changing from one number to the next either reduces light transmission or increases light transmission by a factor of two. This mathematical method of computing light transmission is obviously based on the assumption that the lens is perfect and that there is no light loss from internal reflections (flare) or absorption by the glass. For practical purposes this is true, except when the aperture of the lens approaches "full aperture" (i.e. its widest diameter). This defect is minimal with modern lenses and is overcome by through-the-lens metering which measures actual and not the calculated amount of light transmitted by the lens.

However, there is another more serious defect in the relationship between the f-number (aperture) and light transmission. The consistency of the relationship between light transmission and f-number is based on the assumption that the lens is focused on infinity, when, by definition, the distance from the optical center of the lens to the film plane is the focal length of the lens. However, as the lens is focused on subjects nearer than infinity, the lens-film plane distance is increased. When the subject and the image on the film plane are the same size (RR = 1:1), the lens-film plane distance is twice the focal length (i.e. the lens-film plane distance with the lens focused on infinity) (Fig. 3.19). Now it is obvious that in accordance with the inverse square law which states that the intensity of light falls off inversely as the square root of the distance, at RR = 1:1 with the lens-film plane distance being twice that of the focal length, the intensity of light reaching the film plane will be only ¼ of that for the same subject focused at infinity and with the lens set to the same f-number on the lens barrel. Thus, at RR = 1:1, although the lens aperture has not been altered, it is behaving as if it were two f-numbers smaller because it is now passing only ¼ of the light. Thus, a lens set at a marked aperture of f-16 is really behaving as if it were at f-32 at RR = 1:1. The *f*-numbers marked on the lens barrel are called *relative f*-numbers, and these are true only when the lens is focused on infinity.

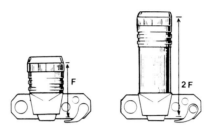

Figure 3.19. At R:R = 1 (i.e. life-size) (*right*), the lens-film plane distance is twice that of the lens focused at infinity (*left*).

In fact, increasing the lens-film distance (i.e. focusing on closer subjects) has little effect on exposure factors until RR = 1:5 or less is reached (Kodak, 1972b) (Table IX). However, the relative *f*-number now behaves as if it were really a smaller relative *f*-number, and that number is really the functional number called the *effective f*-number. The terminology of *relative* and *effective f*-numbers is confusing. An alternative term for *relative f*-number could be *engraved* or *marked f*-number, meaning the number marked on the lens barrel. *Effective f*-number is relatively unambiguous. The really important value is the *effective f*-number because it is an absolute value indicating light transmission in a perfect lens. Thus, *relative* and *effective f*-numbers are identical when the lens is focused on infinity and, in practice, for RR's greater than 1:10. However, for RR's 1:10 to 1:1, the *f*-numbers marked on the lens are incorrect, and now their effective aperture must be used in the calculation of exposure. All of this simply means is that if exposure is standardized for an RR (say 1:4) at *f*-19 (marked on the camera), exposure correction factors, variously called "close-up exposure factors" or "bellows factors," have to be applied to correct the exposure at other RR's. The methods for doing this are frequently confusing and disconcerting.

There are basically three methods of correcting the exposure for these close-up factors.

1. After selecting the aperture from the exposure table (Table IX), calculate the *effective f*-number at the RR used. To compensate for the exposure factor:
   a. select a slower shutter speed
   b. open the aperture by the amount of the exposure factor

Table IX
**CLOSE-UP EXPOSURE FACTORS AND EFFECTIVE APERTURES EQUIVALENT TO *f*-19
AT RR'S 1:10–1:2**

RR	Exposure Factor	Fraction of f-Stop Equivalent to Exposure Factor	Relative Aperture (f-number)* Equivalent to an Effective Aperture of f-19	
			Actual	Approximate
1:10	1.21×	1/3	17.3	16
1:9	1.23×	1/3	17.1	16
1:8	1.26×	1/3	16.8	16
1:7	1.3×	1/3	16.6	16
1:6	1.36×	1/2	16.3	16
1:5	1.44×	1/2	15.8	16
1:4	1.55×	2/3	15.2	16
1:3	1.77×	5/6	14.2	14
2:5	1.96×	1	13.5	13.4
1:2	2.25×	1 1/6	12.6	12.5
1:1	4×	2	9	9

NOTE: This table shows the increase in exposure required at different RR's and the relative apertures equivalent to an effective aperture of f-19 at those RR's. With our equipment, the exposure for an average subject illuminated by two lamps is 1/8 second at an effective aperture of f-19 using Kodachrome 40 film. This table allows the photographer to select the relative aperture, i.e. the one marked on the camera's lens barrel or aperture ring, equivalent to an effective aperture of f-19, for RR's between 1:10 and 1:1.

*The relative aperture is the f number marked on the lens. The numbers of full, half and third stops are listed in Table VIII.

2. Calculate or select from a table the *relative* aperture (marked aperture) of the lens that now corresponds to the desired *effective f*-number. Thus, by reference to Table IX, an *effective* aperture of f-19 at RR = 1:4 is obtained by using the marked (*relative*) aperture of f-15. From Table IX it will be seen that this is only 1/6 stop from f-16 and therefore no significant error is incurred if the marked aperture of f-16 is used.

The methods 1a and 1b are the ones usually listed in most photographic books, but they are very difficult to apply accurately. The shutter speed can usually only be doubled or halved. Thus, changing shutter speed cannot be used to make most of the corrections (Table IX) and can be used accurately only at RR = 1:1 where a 4X exposure is required.

The other method (see 2 above) is to calculate the *effective f*-number of a marked aperture such as f-16. At RR = 1:4, this will be equal to $(1 + M) \times f$-16 = f-20. The convention is to use this formula in which M = magnification which is identical to RR. Thus, to correct this, the aperture will have to be opened by a little more than a half stop (Table IX). This method has even more potential for miscalculation (e.g. at RR = 1:2 the close-up exposure factor is 2.5X). This means opening the aperture by about 1-1/4 stops.

The simplest alternative is to standardize *effective* apertures. Ours are *f*-19 for average subjects illuminated by two lights and *f*-13 when one light is used (Table VII). Thus the question is, "Which *relative* (marked) aperture on the lens barrel is equivalent to *f*-19 or *f*-13 at the RR used?" This can be calculated from the formula:

$$\text{effective } f\text{-number} = (1 + M) \times \text{relative } f\text{-number}$$

In this case, by transposition, the formula is changed so that:

$$\text{relative } f\text{-number} = \frac{\text{effective } f\text{-number}}{1 + M}$$

Thus to select the *relative* (marked) aperture equivalent to an *effective* aperture of *f*-19 and RR = 1:4, these values are substituted in the above equation to obtain a value of *f*-15. As stated above, this is close to *f*-16, and the *f*-16 aperture marked on the lens barrel should be selected to obtain an *effective* aperture of *f*-19 at RR = 1:4. However, rather than having to do this calculation at the time of taking the photograph, a table can be constructed (Table X) using the above formula and Table VI, which lists numerical values of full, half and one-third relative apertures.

Only the full stops (Table VIII) are marked on the camera lens, and the positions of half stops are usually shown by a dot, detent or click stop. Third stops are unmarked and their position has to be estimated in relation to the half-stop positions. Most modern cameras have equal spacing between full-stop numbers engraved on the aperture ring. This is convenient. Older lenses had progressively (geometrically) shorter distances between full-stop markings as *f*-22 was approached. Some lens had only 1–3 mm between the positions of *f*-11, *f*-16 and *f*-22, and half and third stops could not be selected accurately or, in some cases, at all. The spacing between engraved full stops and the presence or absence of detent at the half stops between *f*-11, *f*-16 and *f*-22 (the apertures most commonly used with specimen photography) should be considered when selecting a lens.

In practice, it is easy to use the standardized exposure tables (Tables VII and X) once the RR in use is known. The RR may either be read off the lens barrel or calculated by measuring the width, in inches, of the field in focus of a 35mm camera. The number of inches of the ruler is

Table X
SPECIMEN PHOTOGRAPHY
STANDARD EXPOSURES FOR KODACHROME 40 FOR LENS
WITHOUT AUTOMATICALLY COMPENSATING DIAPHRAGM
Average Subject at $^1/8$ Second

RR	f-*Stop With 2 Lamps**	f-*Stop with 1 Lamp*
> 1:10	19 ($^1/2$ stop between *f*-11 and *f*-16)	13.5 ($^1/2$ stop between *f*-11 and *f*-16)
1:10–1:4	16	11
1:3	14 (close down $^2/3$ stop from *f*-11)	10 (close down $^2/3$ stop from *f*-8)
2:5	13.5 ($^1/2$ stop between *f*-11 and *f*-16)	9.6 ($^1/2$ stop-between *f*-8 and *f*-11)
1:2	12.6 (close down $^1/3$ stop from *f*-11)	9 (close down $^1/3$ stop from *f*-8)

Light subjects such as whole fixed brain . . . . close $^1/2$ stop.
Very light subject such as slices of formalin fixed bleached brain . . . . close 1 stop.
Dark subjects such as liver . . . . open $^1/2$ stop.
Black subjects such as Angus hide . . . . open 1 stop.

*Colotran Multi-6 lamps with 650W bulbs, 42 inches from the subject.

approximately the denominator of the RR, because the 35mm frame is approximately 1 inch wide. Thus, if 4 inches are visible across the width in the principal plane of focus, the RR = 1:4. Then, by referring to Table IX, it is possible to determine which aperture marked on the lens is equivalent to an *effective* aperture of *f*-19. If the RR is between the RR's listed in the table, then the *relative* aperture will have to be estimated. Once the relative aperture has been set, then the usual corrections for reflectivity of the specimen, if it is darker or lighter than average, can be made.

There is another reason for selecting the *effective* aperture rather than increasing the exposure time. Unless the exposure is corrected by opening the diaphragm from the *relative* (marked) aperture, as opposed to the alternative of increasing exposure time, a marked aperture such as *f*-16 at RR = 1:2 is really optically an *effective* aperture of *f*-27 which may cause loss of resolution (Table V). *Thus, close-up exposure factors should be used to open the aperture of the lens and not to increase the length of exposure time by choosing a slower shutter speed.* Also, in the standardized exposure technique we recommend with our equipment, the shutter speed is kept at $^1/8$ second. This eliminates one variable. If exposure times are increased, this can result in exposures becoming so long as to cause reciprocity failure. In the case of RR = 1:2, the exposure increase is from $^1/8$ second to $^1/4$ second, the closest shutter speed to give an exposure increase of

2.25X (Table IX). Additional correction would have to be made by opening the aperture. However, this exposure time would cause reciprocity failure with some Kodak color films resulting in color casts and slight underexposure and the *effective* aperture at *f*-27 would also reduce resolution. All of these factors would decrease the quality of the photograph.

Exposure factors have to be considered with all lenses used at RR's < 1:10 except those which use supplementary lenses (usually screwed or pressed onto the front of the camera's lens) to increase the RR, provided the camera's lens is still focused on infinity. There is one exception. In the late 1960s, Nikon fitted 50mm *f*-3.5 Micro-Nikkor lenses (numbers 220,000 to 273,000) with an automatically compensating diaphragm (Fig. 1.11). This mechanism opened or closed the lens' aperture so that the lens always transmitted the same amount of light at the same *relative* *f*-number from infinity to RR = 1:2. In other words, the engraved or *relative f*-number remained the *effective f*-number from infinity to RR = 1:2. This type of lens is invaluable, as it does away with the annoyance and frustration of making adjustment to the exposure to correct for close-up factors. In practice, these adjustments are easy to forget or to miscalculate. The compensating diagram has been discussed further under "Camera."

The objective of all this standardization is to minimize the time taken to illuminate, focus, compose and expose photographs of specimens and thus to prevent specimens drying out. The idea of keeping the camera's shutter speed constant has been recommended by Smialowski and Currie (1960a) who used a 1/4 second with their equipment. By keeping the shutter speed constant and using a lens which does not need adjustment for "close-up factors" at RR's less than 1:10, the photographer is able to concentrate on lighting, framing and composing the picture, as the only adjustment to the camera is to set the aperture from the exposure table (Table VII). We routinely take three exposures, simply because it is cheaper than having duplicates made. Exposures are bracketed over 1/2 stop (e.g. from *f*-16–*f*-19) for a subject which has average reflectance but has some dark areas. If the subject tends to be lighter than normal or have some lighter areas, the exposures are made from *f*-19 to *f*-22. Exposure repeatability has been excellent. The latitude of Kodachrome 40 film helps, but with specimens such as fixed bleached brain slices which are completely white, the latitude for optimal results is only about 1/3 of a stop.

The beginner will probably feel more secure to use lights in their standardized positions. Once confidence has been gained, he can experiment with the amount of fill-in light needed to illuminate the specimen optimally. This departure from the standardized positions does not complicate exposure estimation significantly. The difference in exposure between using one and two lamps is 1 stop, from f-13 to f-19 for the average subject. Therefore, if the amount of fill-in light is reduced (e.g. by moving the fill-in lamp further away in order to enhance texture or modeling), the exposure will still lie between f-13 and f-19. It is therefore most likely it will be approximately f-16. Therefore, by bracketing over half a stop, correct exposure is easily obtained. After little experience, estimation of the exposure is easy.

Exposure Standardization for Black-and-White Films

The procedure used for standardizing exposures for color films can be applied to black-and-white films, also. Slow films, such as Kodak Panatomic X or Efke (Adox) KB-14, are used. Black-and-white films have far more exposure latitude than color films, and because correct exposure and development are difficult for the inexperienced to judge, evaluation of the negatives should be made by a trained photographer who is competent to evaluate density and contrast and also print the negatives. Once the correct exposures have been determined, a table of exposures (Table XI) can be devised. Black-and-white 35mm film is relatively cheap, and thus it is better to take several exposures of the same subject, bracketing exposures by plus or minus one to two stops. Because the photographer is not preoccupied with determining exposure, he can experiment with the lighting by rotating the specimen in relation to the modeling light and varying the amount of fill-in illumination. These are critically important steps in black-and-white photography.

Flash Exposure

Correct exposure with flash units can be obtained by four methods.

1. Calculated or standardized for specific RR's.
2. Automatic flash units with a sensor mounted either on the flash head or on the camera lens or body.
3. Dedicated flash units which control exposure by sensors in the camera body.
4. Calculation of exposure from a flash meter.

Table XI
SPECIMEN PHOTOGRAPHY
STANDARDIZED EXPOSURES FOR KODAK PANATOMIC X AND EFKE KB-14 FILMS

Subject	No. of Lamps*	Shutter Speed	Aperture
Average	2	$1/4$ sec.	f-16
Average	1	$1/2$ sec.	f-16
Fixed bleached brain slice	1	$1/4$ sec.	f-16
Black haired skin	1	$1/2$ sec.	f-11
		or 2 sec.**	f-16

*Colortran Multi-6 lamps with 650W bulbs, 42 inches from the subject.

**At speeds of 1 second or longer, Kodak black-and-white films require adjustment for reciprocity failure. An exposure of 2 seconds is required at an indicated exposure of 1 second (Kodak, 1984b).

Shaw (1984) recommends that flash exposures be "managed" (i.e. calculated and standardized) rather than the operator relying on automatic or dedicated units. Presumably, this is because flash sensors, like exposure meters, are calibrated on the assumption that subjects are "average." Sensors for automatic units are incorporated either into the flash head itself, or are "remote" with the sensor attached to the camera body or lens hood and connected to the flash unit by a cord. This latter arrangement allows the flash unit to be moved off the camera to obtain better modeling, but the sensor controlling the duration of the flash is still mounted where it can monitor the light received by the lens. Our automatic unit, used with the Nikon f-3.5 Micro-Nikkor lens with an automatically compensating diaphragm, has produced reasonably reliable results with cadaver photography so long as direct reflections from stainless steel tables or shiny surfaces are avoided. Sensors make no adjustment for close-up exposure factors to compensate for a change in *effective f*-number when RR's less than 1:10 are used. A lens with an automatically compensating diaphragm and "dedicated" flash units avoid this problem. Shaw (1984) points out that most sensors read a large area and like all exposure meters they assume that the subject is "average" and reflects 18 percent of the light falling on it, and thus are mislead by very light or very dark subjects.

Many dedicated flash units also control the duration of flash by remote sensors, but these are mounted in the camera and read light reflected from the film plane. Thus, they have the advantage of monitoring only the area seen by the camera's lens. However, again, they assume that the subject has average reflectance and convert all subjects into mid-grey tones. White feathers will be darkened and black skin lightened. The only way the operator can compensate for this departure in average reflectance is to change the ISO (ASA) number on the camera. In our experience, exposure control with TTL–OTF metering has been excellent except in the case of very light or very dark subjects.

If automatic units are not used, the alternative is to calculate or standardize exposures for specific RR's. This is the procedure used by McGavin (1961a, 1961b), which is described under "Special Senses, Eye." Flash exposures were standardized for specific RR's, and to maintain even illumination, the angle of the flash bracket was changed for each RR. Despite the addition of extension tubes, there was relatively little change in exposure. Shaw (1984) also found "that exposure remained constant" as extension tubes were added. Although the *relative* aperture, say f-11, remains constant as the RR becomes smaller, the *effective* aperture really becomes smaller. The working (lens-subject) distance also becomes smaller with the result that the flash-subject distance is reduced. The effect of these two factors, the smaller *effective* aperture and the increased intensity of illumination because of the reduced flash-subject distance, is to cancel each other out and the correct (*relative*) marked aperture remains constant. This is true only if a lens *without* an automatically compensating diaphragm and if the flash tube and the front lens rim remain in the same position relative to each other. Thus, this requires that as the lens is focused forward, either with its own helical mount or by the addition of extension tubes, the flash tube also has to be moved forward (Shaw, 1984). Shaw (1984) recommends that the flash tube be positioned directly above the front rim of the lens by a custom-made bracket. He also found that the *relative* (marked) lens aperture to give correct exposure remained constant only for RR's of 1:6 and less which are equivalent to field sizes of 6 × 9 inches and smaller. The *relative* aperture to give correct exposure at different RR's has to be found by experiment for each camera-flash unit combination. In many cases, the aperture will remain constant over a range of RR's. However, if it does not, a table similar to the ones constructed by McGavin (1961a, 1961b) can be made.

RECORDS

In our photography room we keep separate accession books for each of the three cameras, one for each of the two vertically mounted cameras loaded with transparency and monochrome film, respectively, and one for the hand-held camera with electronic flash. Samples of these blanks are illustrated in Figures 3.20 and 3.21. There is always a strong element of personal preference in these forms, and most people prefer to design their own. Forms for human specimens have space for type of specimen, provisional diagnosis, patient's name, sex, date and accession number. For veterinary specimens we include the accession number, species, organ, diagnosis, and the pathologist's name. Record sheets should have columns for all of the photographic variables: number of lights used, which light (left or right), type of light (spot or diffused), polarization, shutter speed, aperture, RR and type of background (Fig. 3.20). Separate sheets are used for each specimen. When the 2 × 2 slides are returned from the processing laboratory, those belonging to each pathologist are easily identified and forwarded along with the appropriate record sheet. Incorrect entries are rare and when they do occur the diagnosis and organ described on the log sheets makes identification and correction easy. Another alternative is described by White (1970) who kept track of details of office dermatologic photographs by dictating the information into a small portable tape recorder.

Adhesive labels for the mounted 2 × 2 slides are typed with accession number, species, organ and diagnosis. Ruled blank sheets which indicate the number of spaces available on the label, illustrated in Figure 3.22, are extremely useful, as they allow easy planning of the text for the label without exceeding the label's useful capacity.

SUMMARY OF PHOTO-TECHNIQUE FOR GROSS SPECIMENS

Before each photographic session, check that:

1. Light stands are exactly in designated places. Black spots or arcs can be marked on the floor to indicate the center of the stand.
2. Lights are angled correctly to illuminate the specimen table evenly.
3. Barn doors are closed sufficiently to reduce extraneous light but not to cause uneven illumination on the specimen table.
4. Glass tops of light and black boxes are scrupulously clean.

Before photography of each specimen:

1. Transfer the specimen from the dissection table to the photographic background, placing the specimen in its correct anatomical position with minimal contamination of the background. Avoid

PHOTOGRAPHIC RECORD

GROSS SPECIMEN - FLASH UNIT - EKTACHROME 200

Pathology No. _____   Date _____   Pathologist _____

Camera Counter No.	Species	Organ, Diagnosis	f stop in red square on back of flash unit	Lens - 55 or 105 mm	Shutter Speed	Aperture

Figure 3.20. Accession sheet used for recording details of flash photography of cadavers and organs *in situ.*

    sliding or moving specimens, as this smears the background, particularly glass, which is difficult to clean.

2. Place specimens oozing blood or fluid on paper towels on top of the glass.

3. Frame, compose and focus using a low level of illumination such as room lights or photographic lights with reduced output. This is to prevent specimens drying out (Anon., 1942). Full illumination from the photographic lights will dry specimens. Turn on photographic lamps for a minimal period to check illumination, modeling, shadows and specular highlights. Take the photograph immediately.

4. When texture is important, use only one light, usually the left (60°) main light. If shadows are too deep, use two lights or one lamp and a reflector fill-in. Use either one main light at 60° or a texture light at 75°–80° to illuminate slices of brain and lung or exterior organs with nodular surfaces. Two lights are needed to illuminate deep cavities such as the abdominal or thoracic cavities.

5. If the image is not optimal because of the location of shadows,

GROSS SPECIMEN RECORD - KODACHROME 40

Pathology No. _____   Date _____   Pathologist _____

Camera Counter No.	Species	Organ, Diagnoses	Background Black Box	Background Grey Box	Lamps Left, Right or Both	Lamps Flood, Intermediate or Spot	Shut-ter Speed	Relative (= marked) Aperture (f)

Because the effective aperture remains constant with the Nikon lens with the automatically compensating diaphragm, the RR column can be deleted. However the RR must be recorded with all other lenses otherwise the effective aperture and thus the true exposure cannot be determined. This is highly desirable to trace the origin of faults in exposure. Some users may like to have an additional column for "effective aperture".

Figure 3.21. Accession sheet used for recording details of photography of gross specimens with standardized lamps.

specular highlights or poor modeling, rotate the background and along with it the specimen over an arc of about 45° clockwise and counterclockwise and see if changes in lighting angle improve the rendition of the specimen. Once the best lighting position has been found, rotate the camera back to align it to frame the specimen correctly.

6. Insert 1cm of a ruler at the bottom right-hand corner and an identification label (if necessary) in the bottom left corner. Elevate both of these to the correct plane of focus by using wooden blocks or modeling clay.

7. Select the exposure from the exposure table on the wall (Table VII).

8. Make exposure correction for the RR (Table IX). Select the marked aperture on the lens equivalent to an effective aperture of the average subject (Table X).

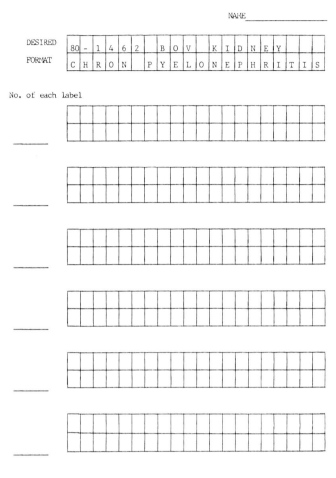

Figure 3.22. Blank used to request labels for 2 × 2 slides. The maximum numbers of letters and spaces are clearly indicated.

9. Make allowance for the reflectivity of the specimen, i.e. darker or lighter than average.
10. Take three exposures over a half-stop range.
11. Record data on the "Photographic Record" sheet.

This system works well. However, it does so only because of cooperation among colleagues. If transparencies are not returned or if the wrong film is loaded into the camera or films are incorrectly loaded onto the take-up spool, confidence in the system is lost. This results in an "every man for himself" attitude. Film is wasted merely because individuals will finish a roll rather than leave it to be handled by another. The only difficulties that have arisen over the years have been in maintenance of the camera. Defects include smears on the lens and viewfinder and occasionally fine debris such as dust and pieces of film in the film chamber. Lens and viewfinders are easily cleaned by cotton-tip swabs after breathing on the lens. To prevent dust and film chips falling onto the lens and shutter, dust is blown out of the camera's film chamber by canned compressed gas after each roll of film is removed, taking extreme care not to direct the jet onto the focal plane shutter which can be damaged by a strong blast. Alternatively, a rubber syringe can be used to blow out the debris.

Chapter 4

SPECIMEN PREPARATION
AND PHOTOGRAPHIC TECHNIQUE

Cooperation between scientists and biological or medical photographers is the optimal arrangement for photography of gross specimens. Each should have an appreciation of the other's role. The pathologist, anatomist or biologist has the responsibility for dissection and
presentation of the specimen in its anatomically correct position, and the
photographer has the responsibility for photographing the specimen so
that the lesions are correctly recorded.

Although such cooperation is optimal, it is relatively rare, and even
well-staffed institutions cannot justify long waiting times by the photographer, particularly when sequential photographs of dissections are to be
taken. There are several alternatives:

1. Specimens can be held in a color preserving solution (discussed
   below). The advantages of this approach have been listed by Williams
   (1984) as convenience of postponing photography, greater east of
   preparing the specimens for photography, simplified lighting and
   highlight control, and (in some cases) tissue structures may be seen
   more clearly. The photography of a batch of specimens at one
   session has been described in detail by Vetter (1984). This procedure makes for optimal use of the photographer's time and, in
   many cases, the pathologist can dissect the specimen free of the
   pressures of necropsy. There are severe penalties. Color-preserving
   solutions do not maintain natural color. Some colors, particularly
   reds, are falsified and rendered more garish, while those due to
   bile and bilirubin are lost. Exudates are washed away or altered in
   character. Specimens will not be optimal for photography, although
   photographs of sequential stages of dissection will be possible.
2. In pathology laboratories without the services of a trained biological photographer, photography has to be done either by the pathologist or the necropsy room technician. Unless acceptable results are

143

obtained in the majority of cases, disappointment will result in an attitude that the whole procedure is not worth the time. Film will be wasted because extra photographs will be taken "in case the others don't come out," and less care may be taken in the dissection because the photographs do not justify the time spent anyway.

Therefore, photographic techniques should be:

1. Highly reliable.
2. The results should justify the expense of the equipment, film and particularly the time to dissect the specimen. With modern photographic equipment, careful standardization and a knowledge of the important factors in this type of photography, it is possible for relatively untrained people to take acceptable color transparencies of many pathological specimens (Vetter, 1969).
3. The optimal compromise is for the necropsy room staff to be able to photograph routine specimens themselves, but be able to refer complicated specimens to the biological photographer. This will mean that sometimes he will have to come to the necropsy room immediately, and sometimes specimens may be held in a color-preserving solution to await his convenience.

Because the final responsibility for the photograph rests with the biological or medical photographer, it is inevitable that many publications on gross specimen photography deal chiefly with the photographic aspects and relatively little with the preparation of the specimens (Smialowski and Currie, 1960a; Hansell and Ollerenshaw, 1962; Kodak, 1966). Observations at meetings confirm that the major defects in transparencies are specimen preparation, dissection and orientation, rather than photography. Support of this view is given by Vetter (1950), who states that "many photographs can be made of gross specimens without undue effort on the pathologist's or photographer's part, at reasonable cost and excellent demonstration of the pathology involved." If the pathologist does not supply suitable specimens, the final result may be an excellent photograph of an unsuitable specimen, the extreme example being the picture described by Hansell (1946) that "conveyed no information save that of a tangled mass of remains." The specimen must be prepared with the lesions highly visible, as it is unlikely that they will be more obvious in the photograph than they are to the naked eye. Selection of specimens for photography should not be an afterthought made after organs and tissues have been contaminated by blood or exudates, sampled for histological and microbiological examinations and even compressed between finger and thumb to test friability. Here the advice of Pulvertaft (1950) for ensuring the best museum specimen applies: "Necropsies should be neither hurried nor perfunctory . . . [and should take place] as soon as possible after death." Techniques for the optimal presentation of lesions in specific organ systems are frequently described in monographs on autopsy technique and are discussed below under each organ system.

NECROPSY TECHNIQUE

The objective is to dissect the cadaver logically and at the same time produce optimal specimens for examination and, if necessary, photography. Technique must be meticulous and contamination of tissues by blood, feces or exudates prevented. Veterinary pathology has the advantage that many animals are euthanatized and the pathologist has the opportunity to prepare the cadaver for optimal presentation of the lesion. Exsanguination is extremely desirable. Blood volume varies from 6 percent to 9 percent of body weight in different species (Swenson, 1977), and the removal of blood results in better visibility of many lesions by preventing hypostatic congestion and also eliminating troublesome oozing of blood from organs. Because thoroughbred horses in training have the highest blood volume as a percentage of body weight, exsanguination in their case is particularly desirable. T_{61}® (American Hoechst Corp. Somerville, NJ 08876), a common euthanasia agent, contains a general anesthetic, a muscle relaxant and a local anesthetic. It frequently stops the heart and thus is not as suitable for exsanguination as conventional barbiturate anesthetics. The desirable procedure is to induce anesthesia to a deep plane to prevent all pain perception and then exsanguinate the animal as rapidly as possible. In large animals, both common carotid arteries should be opened, with care being taken not to incise the trachea. In small animals, the axillary, femoral or carotid arteries may be transected. If exsanguination is not rapid, deep agonal breathing may induce pulmonary artifacts, especially in bovine animals where interstitial pulmonary emphysema is a common sequela. It is essential that the prosector raise the nose of the animal to prevent aspiration of blood, water or regurgitated gastric contents during respiration.

Important factors in necropsy technique are:

1. **Meticulousness.** For example, ribs should be cut neatly, by sharp double-action rib shears. When sectioning organs, the slice must be made using a sharp, straight-bladed knife which is sufficiently long to complete the cut in one motion. The knife should be drawn, not pressed or thrust into the tissues (Mallory and Wright, 1918). To-and-fro cutting produces serrations which are visible and distracting.

2. **Contamination of Specimens.** Contamination must be avoided by careful technique:

   a. Touch tissues as little as possible, as touching can result not only in contamination but digital pressure from gloves can cause depressions on the surface of a specimen such as a liver or cyst.

   Use the so-called "no touch" technique which is really the dissection of tissues using forceps and not the hands to avoid contamination of organs by blood, ingesta, bile, etc. Once the surface of an organ has been contaminated, it can never be completely restored to the original state. Attempt to remove all blood by dabbing gently with soft lint-free paper towels or cloth but not with cotton wool (Martin, 1953) which leaves fibers. Only if absolutely necessary, flush with physiological saline or Jores' solution, as this will increase specular highlights on serous surfaces. Frequently, bile stains cannot be removed. If the surface has a fibrinous exudate, then removal of extraneous blood will alter the appearance of the fibrin. Thus, there is no substitute for meticulous technique which implies use of scrupulously clean gloves and instruments, the "no touch" technique and placing organs on a clean area, preferably on a side table separate from the necropsy table, for dissection.

   b. Never wash organs with water. Endocardium and gastrointestinal mucosa are exceptions, but even they have less specular highlights and brighter colors if unwashed. Water changes the color of some tissues (e.g. serosa such as the liver capsule becomes grey and dull), and water causes hemolysis and thus diffuse pink stains. Pulvertaft (1950) stated that one of the commonest causes of inferior specimens is contact with tap water. If tissues must be washed, use physiological saline or Jores' solution, although the latter can increase the intensity of reds so that all tints of red become similar.

   c. Place organs on paper towels to soak up the blood before placing them on the photographic background. This is not always completely successful, as oozing can continue. Exsanguination is to be preferred.

3. **Removal of Organ Systems En Bloc.** For example, remove the whole

urinary system including kidneys, ureters, urinary bladder (prostate in males) and urethra as a complete system (Fig. 4.46). In carnivores, e.g. dogs, we remove the liver, stomach, duodenum, pancreas and diaphragm in one block to allow examination and display of the bile and pancreatic ducts.

4. **Variations in Standardized Necropsy Techniques.** In a teaching institution it is advantageous in training students to have a standardized necropsy procedure. Thus, in our laboratory, most domestic animals are laid on their right sides, primates and birds on their backs, and horses and elephants on their left sides. For optimal presentations of lesions, it will sometimes be necessary to depart from standardized techniques. For example, because the reticulum is on the left side of the abdomen, the peritoneal adhesions and pericarditis in bovine reticulo-pericarditis will be visible *in situ* once the lateral abdominal wall is reflected, only if the body is laid on its right side. Similarly, dorsal laminectomy to reveal the spinal cord will destroy the laminae and vertebral articular surfaces. If these have lesions and need to be preserved, the spinal cord should be removed by some other technique, e.g. by a ventral approach.

5. **Interim.** The interval between death and photography, and particularly the period between exposure of the tissues or organs at necropsy and photography, must be kept to an absolute minimum. Delay at this point causes loss of "bloom." Fibrinous exudates lose their texture and become amorphous in 5 to 10 minutes after exposure to air and therefore it is essential to photograph lesions such as fibrinous pleurisy or fibrinous pericarditis immediately. Delays can result in other postmortem changes such as hypostatic congestion, hemolysis, hemoglobin imbibition and rigor mortis. For optimal results, where possible, animals should be euthanatized by exsanguination under deep anesthesia. The removal of blood prevents the obscurring of lesions and also prevents oozing from cut surfaces.

Specimens awaiting photography should not be allowed to dry. If a delay is unavoidable, there are several alternatives.

  a. Cover specimens on a tray with paper towels moistened (not wet) with physiological saline, either at room temperature or in the refrigerator.
  b. Place the specimen in physiological saline solution.
  c. Place the specimen in a color preservative solution. (Generally, (a) is to be preferred for brief delays. The advantages and disadvantages of color preservatives are discussed below.)

INFECTION CONTROL

Martin (1953) states that all human autopsy material should be considered infective and that it is the responsibility of the pathologist to indicate infectivity of the specimen on the photography request form. In a veterinary necropsy laboratory, the most dangerous specimens are those infected with diseases transmissible to man, but it is also necessary to prevent the spread of animal pathogens outside the necropsy room. It is wisest to assume that all material is infective with the exception of fixed tissues, tissues from gnotobiotic animals and some laboratory animals used in toxicity trials. At the University of Tennessee's veterinary necropsy laboratory, we have seen over a dozen different diseases transmissible from animals to man in animals sent to necropsy. The most dangerous were rabies, psittacosis, tularemia and yersiniosis. Highly infectious materials such as monkey herpes infections and organisms that are difficult to kill, such as anthrax spores, are best not moved into the photography room.

Routine Photographic Procedures for Infective Material. Contamination of cameras during photography of autopsy specimens is a real problem. LeBeau (1973) cultured *Staphylococcus aureus* from the focusing ring and cable release of the camera used to photograph specimens from a human autopsy case of *Staphylococcus aureus* pneumonia. The same organism was recovered from the glass specimen plate. The photographer can become infected by touching infectious specimens, contaminated equipment or possibly by aerosols produced by the photographic lamps drying out the specimen or exudates (Williams, 1984). One common cause of contamination of photographic equipment is an overly long cable release which can touch the specimen at very close working distances. If equipment becomes contaminated, it should be wiped clean with a disposable sponge or wipe moistened in germicide and then sponged again with germicide. LeBeau (1973) recommends a variety of these including povidone iodine (75–150 ppm), quaternary ammonium compounds (0.2%–1%) and o-phenyl phenols (2.5%).

Specimens should be touched only with gloved hands and gloved hands should touch only the specimen or its background, never photographic equipment. To develop desirable habits, it is wisest to take the same basic precautions with all specimens. It helps if there are two persons to do the photography, a "clean" person to focus and frame the camera and to record the data, and a gloved prosector to handle and orient the specimen. If only one person is present, one solution is for the operator to use one gloved hand to orient the specimen and a clean hand to operate the camera and lights. The highest form of professional callousness is for a pathologist or a photographer to contaminate photographic equipment. The author knows of one person who routinely contaminated equipment without consideration for his colleagues but wore gloves to protect himself. Such action is not only reprehensible but it destroys confidence in the safety of the system.

Handling of infectious specimens is made easier if there are well-defined "clean" and "dirty" counters in the photography room (Fig. 1.2). We have a stainless steel dissection counter and a clean counter for records and camera accessories. After photography, paper towels and swabs are incinerated or autoclaved, and counter-tops and photographic backgrounds are cleaned and disinfected. If the specimen is extremely dangerous, then the photographic backgrounds are autoclaved even if this results in damage. All exudates dropped on the floor are swabbed, cleaned and disinfected. This is a good reason for the photography room to have an impervious concrete floor with floor drains.

Some color-preserving solutions (e.g. Jores') were once regarded as fixatives and capable of killing pathogens, but these solutions contain so little formalin that they do not even fix well, much less guarantee the sterilization of pathogenic bacteria such as mycobacteria.

Highly Infectious Cases. If there is no danger from aerosol infection, a specimen of highly infectious material can be prepared under a hood, placed on a disposable or autoclavable photographic background in a stainless steel tray, covered with saline moistened paper towels and transferred to the photography room. Here the specimen should be photographed quickly, and then the specimen, background, tray, instruments and gloves discarded into the autoclave. This procedure is also suitable for specimens infected with diseases such as tularemia, psittacosis or mycobacteriosis, provided certain precautions are taken to prevent aerosol infection. Air flow should always be downward to carry pathogenic organisms away from the operator's face. Air should enter through ducts located in or close to the ceiling and be exhausted close to the wall-floor junction (Fig. 1.3). Also, a long focal length lens such as a 105mm macro-lens should be used because its long working distance keeps the operator's face away from the specimen. In close-up photographs of air-sacculitis in a bird with psittacosis, a 55mm macro-lens has a working distance of only 4 to 6 inches, thus increasing the chances of aerosol infection of the photographer. Masks should always be worn, and infectious specimens should never be touched by a bare hand or allowed to touch any photographic equipment.

Laboratories specializing in highly infectious diseases use cameras in waterproof housings that can be disinfected with such agents as hypochlorite (10–2500 ppm), quaternary ammonium compounds (0.2%–1%) and povidone iodine (75–150 ppm) (Kodak, 1972a), or they use cheap equipment that can be discarded into the autoclave after use. Film is sterilized by gas-claving, in most cases by a cycle with 27 inches of vacuum, a relative humidity of 30% to 50% at 130°F (54.4°C) for 2 hours or 4 hours at 100°F (37.8°C). The camera should be wrapped in a polyethylene bag of 3 to 4 mils thickness (Kodak, 1972a).

COLOR RESTORATION AND PRESERVATION

In our experience, nothing can compare with the results obtained when specimens are removed uncontaminated at necropsy, require no washing or blotting and are photographed with minimal delay. This raises the question, What place is there for color preservation or color restoration in photography of specimens? There are two major needs for this:

1. *Photography has to be delayed,* e.g. if complicated specimens require expert photography and the photographer is not immediately available.
2. *Specimens filled with blood,* e.g. splenic hematoma and hemangiomas. Photographs of the exterior of such spleens show the misshapen appearance, but cross sections of a hematoma or hemangiomas are frequently so bloody and ooze so continuously that they reveal little to the naked eye and much less in a photograph. For these, fixation of a slice in 10% formalin or Schein's fixative, followed by "restoration" of color, will produce a useful, although not completely faithful record of the color of the specimen.

Maintenance of color in gross pathological specimens has been attempted for approximately 100 years, chiefly in the preparation of museum specimens. The advantages and disadvantages of many of these methods have been reviewed (Armed Forces Institute of Pathology, 1957). Because it was not always possible to photograph pathological specimens immediately, some of these methods have now been used to either preserve or restore color after fixation for later photography. There is, however, a difference between "color preservation" and "color restoration." In the latter, the color is "lost" during fixation and then "restored" (Armed Forces Institute of Pathology, 1957).

There are considerable arguments about what constitutes "natural color" in an organ or tissue. Thus, at surgery, tissues are filled with circulating blood and frequently appear "congested," while at necropsy, tissues may be congested or pale, depending on such conditions as hypostatic congestion or whether the animal was exsanguinated at euthanasia. However, it must be emphasized that none of the color-preservation or restoration methods actually preserve "natural" color. Subtle differences of color, particularly in the pinks and reds, are lost, a factor which was not important decades ago when color films were unable to record minor variations in color.

This section will discuss the advantages and disadvantages of the various methods, but it must be emphasized that results produced will never equal those obtained with fresh specimens photographed with minimal delay.

Color-Restoration Methods After Formalin Fixation

Methods used include:

1. 80% to 95% ethanol (Bohrod and Beiter, 1944).
2. sodium hydrosulfite, Schein and Wentworth techniques (Armed Forces Institute of Pathology, 1957)
3. antimony trioxide solution (Meiller, 1938)

1. **Ethanol Color Restoration** (Bohrod and Beiter, 1944)

This method has been advocated for photography of eyes which have to be fixed and hardened before they are sliced. The technique can also be used to harden friable, soft and easily distorted tissues which need to be sliced to reveal changes on a cut surface. A disadvantage is that fixation time must be minimal. It is less successful with those tissues containing large quantities of blood. Thus, it is not the method of choice if colored photographs of specimens are required after weeks or months of formalin fixation.

The procedure is:

1. Fix in 10% formalin for as short a time as possible, sufficient only for adequate penetration. Small organs such as eyes require only 24

to 48 hours. The more blood in the tissue, the less tolerance to prolonged fixation.

2. Wash for half to one hour. Fragile specimens may be washed by multiple changes of water; more robust specimens can be washed under running water.

3. Color restoration must be done under constant observation to detect the peak of the color development. Place the tissue in 80% to 95% ethanol and watch until the color reaches a peak, usually in 10 to 30 minutes (Bohrod and Beiter, 1944), although Martin (1953) states that some specimens take up to 2 hours. After reaching the peak of their color, specimens loose their brightness and become pale. Because of this, color restoration should be done with the photographic equipment ready.

Recommendations for Specific Organs

These are (Bohrod and Beiter, 1944):

a. *Large organs.* Because large fixed specimens usually give poor results, fix a 1cm wide slice (e.g. of spleen) for 24 hours (Bohrod and Beiter, 1944). Results with hearts have been mediocre and with lungs poor (Bohrod and Beiter, 1944). Views of the external surface of the kidneys are satisfactory and speckled lesions such as those due to multifocal embolic nephritis are good, although the color may not be true. We have found that with ethanol color restoration, colors on the cut surface of the kidney are distorted so that both cortex and medulla become red, whereas before fixation the medulla was grey.

b. *Brain.* This is frequently difficult to photograph in the fresh state because of its flabby nature. However, meningeal exudates should be photographed immediately, because their color after formalin fixation is not restored well by alcohol. Fix large brains (e.g. human) for 4 to 5 days or longer (Bohrod and Beiter, 1944). In our experience, brains of small domestic animals are fixed and hardened adequately for slicing after 2 to 3 days. Wash, slice transversely and restore the color. Then either keep the cut surface wet with alcohol from a dropping bottle or wash in water. As some specimens become grey after a water wash, the first method is preferred. Alternatively, the brain slices can be photographed under fluid, preferably 95% alcohol (Bohrod and Beiter, 1944). Results are acceptable. Blood vessels are accentuated. Reds are darker than normal with little variation in color saturation in various tissue components.

Restoration of color is probably unnecessary for photography of the majority of brain slices. If brains have been fixed for only several days, their cut surfaces will frequently show color differences. (See details on preparation and photography of brains under "Nervous System" in this chapter.)

   c. *Eyes.* Because eyes have to be processed for histological sections, they are passed through graded alcohols to reduce distortion and shrinkage rather than being put directly from water into 95% alcohol. The technique is to (Bohrod and Beiter, 1944):
   a. Fix for 24 to 48 hours.
   b. Wash half to one hour in running water.
   c. Process through graded alcohols from 50% to 95% ethanol over 24 hours.
   d. Cut a single culotte.
   e. Place in 95% alcohol for several hours to allow hardening.
   f. Section parallel to the first cut.
   g. Photograph under 95% alcohol.
The technique is useful, although the final colors are not really natural. It can be employed to increase tonal contrast in black-and-white photographs. Formalin-fixed lesions with little texture and low contrast are notoriously difficult to photograph in black and white, and restoration of color increases contrast and considerably improves monochrome photographs.

   2. **Sodium Hydrosulfite.** Of the methods reviewed by the Armed Forces Institute of Pathology (1957), the most successful for color fidelity were those of Wentworth and Schein. These restore color with sodium hydrosulfite ($Na_2S_2O_4$, MW = 171.114), also known as sodium sulfoxalate and sodium dithionite. Best results are obtained after fixation with Schein's fixative (Schein, 1951) which is a 5% buffered acid formalin (pH = 6.9) with the following formula:

   4.69 g   sodium phosphate, monobasic, anhydrous, NaH_2PO_4
   5.9 g   sodium phosphate, dibasic, $Na_2HPO_4.H_2O$
   50 ml   37% formaldehyde solution
   1 liter   tap water.

Fixation takes a minimum of two weeks and frequently up to 3 or 4 weeks. Perfusion fixation is desirable. Unfortunately, specimens fixed in unbuffered 10% formalin have reduced capability of color restoration. In an emergency, we have diluted 10% NBF 1:1 with water to give 5% NBF with reasonably good results. Although 10% NBF should be neutral, in fact the pH is often approximately 6.9 and therefore slightly acidic, as is Schein's fixative. Color is restored by the addition of 0.5 grams of powdered hydrosulfite per 100 ml of buffer or per 100 ml of Schein's fixative (buffer + 5% formalin) directly into a closed box. Exposure to air is detrimental to the color as the hydrosulfite is oxidized, causing an irreversible loss of color in the specimen (Armed Forces Institute of Pathology, 1957). The sodium hydrosulfite is difficult to get into solution and can cause the fluid to become cloudy for hours (Armed Forces Institute of Pathology, 1957), a considerable inconvenience. Salthouse (1955) also used hydrosulfite to return specimens to an approximation of their original color after fixation in 10% formalin. However, the solution he used consisted of 0.5 g sodium hydrosulfite in 100 ml of 70% isopropyl alcohol. No other details were given. Pulvertaft (1950) recommends placing the washed fixed specimen in 0.4%–0.6% solution of sodium hydrosulfite solution until the maximum color restoration is obtained.

3. **Antimony Trioxide Solution.** Meiller's (1938) method is considered by Armed Forces Institute of Pathology (1957) to be one of the most effective in restoring color to tissues fixed in 10% formalin. In our experience the reds are harsh and lack any delicacy.

The method is:

1. Fix in 10% formalin. Avoid overfixation. Fix intestine for less than 10 hours and pieces of liver and spleen for less than 24 hours.
2. Wash in running water for 3 to 6 hours.
3. 2% NH_4OH solution for 5 to 10 minutes.
4. Wash in running water for 1 hour.
5. Antimony trioxide solution. Prepare a saturated solution of antimony trioxide in distilled water (about 5 g per liter) and filter. To each 100 ml of filtrate add:

100 g	potassium acetate
100 g	chloral hydrate
50 ml	glycerin

Stir well until chemicals are completely dissolved.

If tissues have been left in fixative for too long, good colors may be obtained by cutting a new surface.

Preservation of Color

In contrast to the color-restoration techniques in which tissues are fixed and bleached and color is later "restored," color is never "lost" with the color-preservation methods. Methods include immersing specimens in:

1. so-called "modified" Jores' or Klotz solutions.
2. antibiotic solution and refrigeration.
3. towels moistened with physiological saline, with or without refrigeration.

1. **So-Called Modified Klotz or Modified Jores' Solution.** These solutions, of which there are several modifications, resemble Klotz-Kaiserling solution (1946) more closely than Jores' (1896), Klotz-MacLachlan (1914) or Klotz and Colburn (1916) (cited by Armed Forces Institute of Pathology, 1957). Their formulae have been summarized in Table XII. The formula popularized by Vetter (1960) is listed under the name "modified Jores'." The exact method of action of these solutions is unclear, and the wide diversity in formulae points to the empirical selection of components. A 1% solution of sodium bicarbonate for washing specimens produces much the same color. We currently omit the chloral hydrate, a relatively expensive and strictly controlled drug. Some institutions wash organs, place them in modified Jores' solution (ratio of 1:10 of specimen to Jores' solution) for 24 to 36 hours and then change the solution (ratio of 1:1 of tissue to Jores' solution) (Vetter, 1960). Modified Jores' solution contains only 2% formalin and fixes to a depth of 1mm to 2mm. Thus, tissue blocks for histopathological examination should be removed at the time of the original dissection or shaved from the surface of Jores' fixed blocks (Vetter, 1960). Dukes (1975) has indicated that both color preservation and fixation can be achieved for 1 to 2 weeks with brains by using modified Jores' solution in which the formalin concentration has been increased to 20 percent. This may work with human brains, but in our experience animal brains are bleached in 1 to 2 days. However, we have noticed that longitudinal cuts of bones with osteogenic sarcoma placed in Jores' solution for 1 to 2 hours have maintained their pink color even after subsequent fixation in 10% NBF for several days.

Because of the falsification of red colors, we have ceased to use modified Jores' solution except for bones and joints waiting for specialized

Table XII
FORMULAS OF JORES' AND KLOTZ' SOLUTIONS

	Jores (1896)*	Klotz & Maclachlan (1915)*	Klotz and Kaiserling (1946)*	Jores' #1 (Schein, 1951)	Modified Jores' (Vetter, 1960)	Modified Jores' #1 (Bridgeman and Hummelbaugh, 1963)	Jores' (Ludwig, 1979d)
Sodium chloride	10g	5.6g	7g	9g	4.5g	9g	10g
Sodium bicarbonate	…	6.2g	4g	10g	8.1g	10g	…
Sodium sulfate dessicated	20g	6.9g	…	11g	10g	11g	20g
Chloral hydrate	…	31.2g	31.2g	50g	18g	50g	…
37% Formalin	50ml–100ml	31.2ml	25.6ml	100ml	20ml	80ml	20ml–40ml
Potassium nitrate	…	11.8g	…	19g	…	…	…
Potassium sulfate	…	0.6g	…	1g	…	…	…
Glycerin	…	…	…	…	…	100ml	…
Magnesium sulfate	20g	…	20g	…	…	…	20g
Water	1000ml	1000ml	1000ml	1000ml	1000ml	1000ml	1000ml
% Formalin	5%–10%	3%	2.5%	10%	2%	8%	2%–4%

*Formula as cited by Armed Forces Institute of Pathology (1957).

photography and when photography of routine specimens is delayed for longer than overnight.

Jores' solution has the following disadvantages:

1. Pinks and reds are quickly converted to a uniform light red, so that subtle differences in color are lost. Pink lungs are quickly converted to a light red. Opps (1934) reported that storage in Jores' Fluid No. 1 over 24 hours resulted in "blending of colors." Jores' No. 1 is similar in composition to "modified Jores'" (Table XII).
2. It is a poor fixative since it contains only 2% formalin and pentrates only 1mm to 2mm.
3. Cost. The solution is relatively economical if commercial grade or grocery store chemicals are used, but chloral hydrate is expensive. Its purpose in the solution is unclear, but it may be antibacterial. We now omit it and store specimens in fresh Jores' solution in a refrigerator.

2. **Antibiotic Solution and Refrigeration.** Lewis and Morton (1963) investigated the storage of surgical specimens in antibiotic solutions. They recommended that the best method was storage in a solution of physiological saline to which 300 mg of neomycin and 40 mg of dequalinium per liter had been added, in an airtight container with all air excluded. Colors were retained for 10 days except for lung and thyroid which lost color rapidly. Autopsy material was unsuitable, presumably due to bacterial contamination. The photographs illustrating the article show remarkable retention of colors, but many of these are changed from those of the fresh state.

3. **Physiological Saline.** For storage for several hours, covering of the specimen with a towel, sponge or lint-free disposable paper towel, moistened in physiological saline, has been the most convenient method (Martin, 1961; Williams, 1984). Disposable paper towels are convenient and, if air is excluded, color changes and drying are minimal, but there is some subtle deterioration. If the waiting period is to exceed several hours, the covered specimen should be refrigerated.

Summary

All of the techniques for color retention and restoration have serious disadvantages. Exudates and bile are washed away, friable masses are dislodged or lose their texture and colors are changed significantly. In the case of soft or friable masses whose cut surface is to be photographed, there is little or no alternative to formalin fixation followed by sectioning and color restoration. Formalin fixation with color restoration in ethanol is easy and adequate for most cases. With routine specimens, the best procedure is to dissect specimens, carefully avoiding spillage of blood and feces so that washing is unnecessary, and to photograph them immediately while they still have their "bloom." This can be done quickly and easily with a standardized photographic unit. Results are excellent in the vast majority of cases. Frequently, a photograph taken immediately with such a unit will produce a good photograph of an excellent specimen. Photography later, after color preservation or restoration, may result in an excellent photograph of a good to poor specimen. In our experience, bones and joints held overnight in modified Jores' solution have some falsification of red colors and some pink staining of cartilage but still remain good specimens. In bones, interest is often in changes in shape or in the texture of the articular cartilage which has relatively little color, and thus storage in Jores' fluid has little deleterious effect.

DISSECTION TECHNIQUE

The following sections describe the dissection and photographic technique for anatomic systems discussed in alphabetical sequence.

Abdominal Cavity

Most domestic animals are necropsied in lateral recumbency. For them, the technique of opening the peritoneal cavity by incising through the abdominal wall from the longissimus dorsi muscle to the xiphoid, parallel and just caudal to the costal arch and then along the linea alba from the xiphoid to the symphysis pubis gives good exposure of viscera and any excess peritoneal fluid. Variations in technique are required for special cases, for example, the incision should be paramedian to miss an umbilical hernia. If peritoneal fluids are greatly excessive, fluid will pour out of the abdomen as it is opened. A flash photograph can be taken to record the excess fluid.

Photographs of the peritoneal cavity are used to illustrate:

1. **Displaced Organs.** For example, intestinal torsions and intussusceptions. If these are visible immediately upon opening the abdomen, they can be photographed without further dissection. However, if they are obscured by intestines, the normal intestine should be dissected free of its mesentery and removed from the peritoneal cavity until only the

affected portion remains. This technique is desirable for animals such as herbivores that have long gastrointestinal tracts.

2. **Dilatations.** Gastric dilatations are usually visible immediately upon opening the abdomen, but dilatation of a segment of gut (e.g. colon) may be fully visible only after normal intestine has been dissected free of its mesentery and removed from the abdominal cavity.

3. **Fluids.** For example, transudates (ascites), exudates (peritonitis), blood (hemoperitoneum), or urine (ruptured bladder). Small amounts of fluids cannot be photographed *in situ,* as they may not be visible until viscera have been removed and inevitably, as small mesenteric vessels are severed during removal of intestines, blood stains the fluid. If it is desired to illustrate the character of peritoneal fluid, it should be aspirated into a clear plastic syringe before the abdomen is opened and the syringe and contents photographed with suitable backlighting to reveal the color and transparency of the fluid.

4. **Peritonitis.** Fibrinous exudates of peritonitis rapidly become amorphous and should be photographed immediately after exposure. In our laboratory, small animals are placed on a black Formica covered board and carried to the photography room and photographed under the vertically mounted camera and standardized lights. Sometimes illumination from only one light is better in bringing out the texture of the fibrin.

5. **Hernias.** To preserve umbilical hernias, incisions should be paramedian rather than midline through the linea alba. Inguinal hernias can be unilateral or bilateral and the midline incision will expose the internal inguinal rings and any contents. If the contents of the hernial sac are extensive, they can be demonstrated dramatically by reflecting the skin and incising the lateral wall of the hernial sac sufficiently to reveal the content *in situ.* A hernia in the inguinal canal on the dependent side will not be revealed until most of the intestines have been freed from the mesentery and removed from the abdomen. To illustrate bilateral hernias, one pathologist removed the ventral abdominal wall, including both inguinal canals and herniated gut, and then photographed them from a dorsal (internal) viewpoint.

6. **Vascular Accidents.** For example, the demonstration of an intestinal infarction. A sequence of photographs is required when the abdomen is opened and after the normal intestines have been removed. Large congested spleens such as those due to splenic torsion are best photographed *in situ* so that their size in the abdomen can be appreciated.

7. **Pelvic Cavity.** The portion of the peritoneal cavity in the pelvis should be exposed by removal of the lateral wall of the pelvis. Saggital cuts are made through the pubis to the obturator foramen, caudally from the obturator foramen through the ischium and by a third cut transversely through the neck of the ilium, cranial to the acetabulum to allow removal of the lateral bony wall of the pelvis (Fig. 4.24). After some minor dissection, lesions such as rectal obstruction due to a prostatic hyperplasia or adenocarcinoma and rectovaginal fistulas will be visible.

Photographs of the *in situ* viscera of *large* domestic animals are usually taken with electronic flash and are less successful because of:

1. **Lighting.** This usually lacks modeling if one flash is used, even if this is held away from the camera. With very large animals illumination may be uneven and flat. This problem has been overcome by the use of two dedicated flash units with exposure controlled by the TTL–OTF meters (Fig. 4.58). These flash units have been described under "Equipment" and are highly recommended for both black-and-white and color photography of *in situ* viscera (see also "Cadaver Photography").

2. **Orientation.** Frequently, two photographs are required, a "long shot" for a general view of the body cavity and orientation and a "close-up" for detail.

3. **Backgrounds.** With large animals the background may be cluttered and the stainless steel necropsy table may be distracting. There is no easy way to overcome these problems, but background can be minimized by selection of a high angle of view and carefully framing with a zoom lens to limit the area of the backgrounds. For further discussion, see "Cadaver Photography."

4. **Distortions.** These occur because of an unsuitable angle of view. Many photographs are taken at too low an angle, resulting in distortion and an obtrusive background. The camera's optical axis should be approximately 90° (normal) to the abdominal wall (Fig. 4.59). To achieve this, a high viewpoint such as that from a 6 ft. to 8 ft. high step-ladder is required (Fritts, 1976).

The secret of successful photography of *in situ* organs of large animals is to include enough anatomical landmarks to allow the viewer to orient himself and yet keep the area of interest large enough for detail to be visible. The electronic flash unit needs to be of sufficiently high output to allow the use of relatively small apertures (e.g. *f*-16) so that depth of field is adequate and ambient illumination does not record on the film.

Also, to achieve some modeling, the flash head must be 30°–50° above and to the side of the camera's optical axis, with the fill-in flash at ¼ power mounted on the camera. Dedicated flash units and cameras read the exposure off the film and have given consistently good exposure control for average subjects (see "Electronic Flash Units" under "Equipment").

Alimentary System

Oral Cavity

In our necropsy technique, the upper skin and buccal mucosa are reflected upwards from a mid-ventral (midsagittal) incision starting from the lip and extending caudally between the rami of the mandibles to the pubis. The symphysis of the mandible is split and the upper ramus removed, revealing the oral cavity, hard and soft palates and pharynx. The tongue, soft palate and pharynx, along with the trachea, esophagus and thoracic viscera, are removed in one block. The isolated tongue and pharynx should be photographed in a vertical (Fig. 4.1) format, because the dorsal surface is being viewed. After removal of the complete lower jaw and disarticulation of the head from the atlas, the hard palate and teeth can be photographed in a vertical format (Fig. 4.2). Lighting should be arranged to produce modeling (e.g. of the transverse ridges in the roof of the mouth). Photographs are required to record such changes as pigmentations (melanosis), cleft palate, neoplasia and changes in, or absence of, teeth.

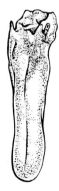

Figure 4.1.

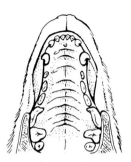
Figure 4.2.

Some lesions in the mouth such as the enlarged tongue of Hurler's disease or a malignant melanoma displacing incisor teeth are best photographed during life. Once the animal is dead and rigor mortis sets in, positioning of the jaws may be difficult. This is particularly true of positioning a dead body to obtain a frontal view of incisors *in situ.*

Teeth

Teeth can be quite difficult to photograph and there are several approaches:

1. **View of the Buccal Surface of the Incisors.** At necropsy these can be photographed nicely by sawing the body of the mandible transversely from the rami. This cut must be exactly transverse so that the specimen will stand vertically on end and require no props which would be visible in the field of view.

2. **Isolated Ramus.** This approach is useful for a lateral (buccal) or medial (lingual) view of the surfaces of the teeth.

3. **Whole Mandible.** In a dorsal view, only the occlusal surfaces of the teeth are visible. A vertically mounted camera does not have the flexibility to obtain optimal views of teeth. An oblique angle which allows viewing of two surfaces (e.g. occlusal and buccal or lingual) appears more realistic as well as allowing the viewer to orient himself easily (Fig. 4.3). As the specimen does not deteriorate rapidly and delay is not important, it can be taken to a specialized photographic studio (see "Skeletal System").

Palate, Hard and Soft

Lesions on the hard palate are visible after one ramus or both rami of the mandible have been removed. However, lesions on the soft palate

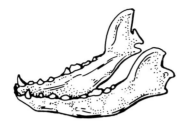

Figure 4.3.

may require further dissection. Preliminary photographs of the palates, viewed from the ventral approach, should be taken. This view is suitable to reveal defects such as cleft palate. However, tumors such as fibrosarcomas and overly long soft palates such as occur in horses are dramatically presented by a midsagittal saw cut through the skull.

Pharynx

Penetrating lesions of the caudal pharyngeal wall, as, for example, those caused by drenching syringes, are difficult to record photographically because orientation is easily lost. These lesions are best photographed after removal of a ramus of the mandible but before removal of the tongue, pharynx and neck organs. It is desirable that a probe such as a rubber catheter be inserted through the puncture site into the area of cellulitis or the sinus which frequently extends down the fascial planes of the neck muscles. Sequential photographs of the dissection should be made. Another approach is to disarticulate the mandible from the skull and then remove the mandible, tongue, pharynx, esophagus and trachea *en bloc.* The pharynx is partially opened by a mid-dorsal incision starting rostrally and a probe is inserted through the site of penetration. Satisfactory photographs of this type of lesion, particularly in black and white, are difficult to make. The site of penetration is usually discolored dark red by cellulitis or medicament and does not have a good color or tonal contrast with the adjacent tissues. Also, the long narrow specimens do not fill the frame and thus both an overall view and a close-up photograph are required.

Tonsils

Photographs of tonsils are usually taken to record enlargement from lymphoid hyperplasia or tumors such as malignant lymphoma or squamous cell carcinoma. After removal of the tongue, pharynx, and neck organs *en bloc,* the dorsal wall of the pharynx should be incised mid-sagittally and retracted laterally to expose the tonsils. This technique gives excellent exposure of the tonsils, the viewer can orient himself easily and lighting from the standardized lamps is excellent (Fig. 4.4).

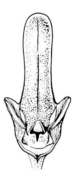

Figure 4.4.

Esophagus

The esophagus is removed *en bloc* with the tongue, neck and thoracic organs. After the pharynx and esophagus have been opened longitudinally along their dorsal midlines, the esophagus can be removed by transecting it near the pharynx, if there are no lesions at that site. Esophageal mucosa is relatively resistant and can be washed gently in cool water without deleterious effect. All tags of fat and fascia projecting beyond the edge of the mucosa should be trimmed off. Also, the incision through the mucosa and muscularis should be neat and relatively straight. This is best accomplished by opening the esophagus along the dorsal midline, with a pair of sharp blunt-nosed scissors, in one gentle continuous motion. After being placed on a photographic background, the mucosa should be stretched gently across its width but not so vigorously as to remove the natural folds.

The vertical format is best, with illumination supplied by one low-placed texture light to the left. This brings out texture of folds, erosions, ulcers and proliferative lesions. Framing and selection of the specimen/background ratio are the most difficult decisions, because the esophagus is long and narrow. Best results are obtained in close-up photographs of small lesions. Photographs of the full length of the esophagus, especially those from large animals, are not successful, as the image of the esophagus is so small that detail is not visible. To reduce the size of the field of view, the esophagus can be arranged in a serpentine fashion or cut in parallel strips. Neither of these alternatives is particularly aesthetically pleasing. When comparison of different portions of the esophagus such as upper cervical and mid-thoracic is required, then parallel segments should be arranged vertically. Each strip of esophagus should be placed with its cranial end to the top of the frame and the segments arranged in order with the most rostral segment to the left and the most caudal to the right.

Some lesions of the eosphagus are best demonstrated with the esophagus *in situ.* These include:

1. Megaesophagus
2. Stomach intussuscepted into the caudal esophagus.
3. Dilatation and obstruction due to a persistent aortic arch.
4. Penetrating foreign bodies, e.g. needle ingested by a cat.
5. Rupture sites, e.g. from intubation.
6. Compression by mediastinal masses, e.g. neoplastic caudal mediastinal lymph node.

Megaesophagus can be difficult to photograph because the dilated flaccid esophagus covered by mediastinum often collapses making the enlargement difficult to discern. The dorsal portion of the overlying lung should be displaced ventrally and the dorsal mediastinum incised to reveal the esophagus. The esophageal dilatation can be redistended by inserting plugs of cotton through an incision in the stomach, but unless this is done with great care, the natural fusiform shape of the dilatation may be lost. A successful photograph will show location, shape, length and diameter of the dilatation.

Photographs of the stomach intussuscepted into the caudal esophagus, esophageal dilatation due to a persistent right aortic arch (Mouwen and deGroot, 1982) and the danger to adjacent organs from foreign bodies penetrating the esophagus can be dramatically depicted with organs *in situ.* Additional photographs of the isolated esophagus can be made later.

Stomach

The stomach of the dog lies to the left with the greater curvature ventrally. Thus, the anatomical position of the isolated unopened stomach in a photograph is with the cardia to the top left, the greater curvature along the left and bottom sides of the frame and the pylorus to the right (Fig. 4.5). This is a caudal view of the stomach and the viewer is easily oriented. If lesions are on the cranial surface of the stomach, the stomach will have to be rotated through 180° on a vertical (dorso-ventral) axis. Display of gastric mucosal lesions is easily done by opening the stomach along the greater curvature from the cardia to the pylorus. If this incision would destroy a lesion, the incision should be displaced slightly towards the lesser curvature. If the contents are of importance (e.g. in hemorrhagic gastritis), the stomach should be placed on a black Formica board and then opened to display the contents. Later, the gastric mucosa should be washed with cool water, blotted lightly with paper towels, placed in its anatomical position and illuminated by one texture light from the left. Results are usually excellent.

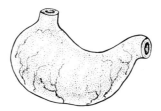

Figure 4.5.

The abomasum of ruminants should be treated similarly, with the greater curvature being placed at the bottom of the frame. Dissection of the rumino-reticulum for the preservation of anatomical relationships and exposure of the mucosa of individual ruminal sacs has been described (McGavin, 1976). In this technique, serosal and fibrous attachments in all grooves on the outside of the rumino-reticulum are manually detached. The rumino-reticulum is laid on its right side and three incisions are made (Fig. 4.6). The first incision (Fig. 4.6, *starred line*) starts on the cranial surface of the reticulum and runs approximately dorso-caudally along the greater curvature to a point, where an extension of the rumino-reticular groove would cross the dorsal greater curvature. The second incision (Fig. 4.6, *dashed line*) extends horizontally from the cranial to caudal grooves, just dorsal to the left longitudinal groove. The third incision (Fig. 4.6, *round dots*) joins the caudal end of the first incision to the cranial end of the second. Because the rumen is subdivided into component sacs, it is difficult to view the whole of its mucosa in one photograph, but by judicious folding much of the mucosa can be exposed for photography. However, for careful examination and photography, the different ruminal sacs must be dissected free. The caudo-dorsal and caudo-ventral blind sacs are removed by cutting completely around their peripheries, cranial to the dorsal and ventral coronary pillars. The caudal pillar remains attached to the ventral sac. The ventral sac is removed from the dorsal sac by cutting just dorsal to the right longitudinal and cranial pillars. As most of the changes in the mucosa will be changes in texture, illumination by a small tungsten-halogen spotlight at approximately 75° to 80° to the lens subject-axis and a photoflood as a fill-in lamp at 45° to the lens subject-axis (Fig. 4.7) (Kodak, 1966) gives excellent results. Photographs of the mucosa of individual sacs of the rumen are taken at half normal size (RR = 1:2). To keep the mucosa flat, because of the limited depth of field at RR's approaching one, the mucosa must be stretched lightly over a flat surface such as a bottle and can be held in place by a rubber band.

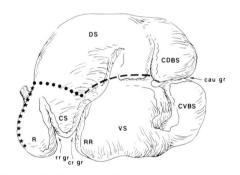

Figure 4.6. Courtesy of *Journal of Animal Science.*

Perforating gastric ulcers appear most realistic when photographed against a black background. A white, grey or colored background visible through the ulcer's orifice appears strange. Perforating ulcers can be accentuated by rubber or colored nylon tubes (Martin, 1953), but, as these can be very distracting, probes should be used only when absolutely essential. A latex rubber catheter is the least distracting probe.

Occasionally, optimal fixation of gastric mucosa and preservation of the shape of the stomach are required. This can be done by placing the stomach in a bath of 10% NBF and distending it with 10% NBF at a pressure of 25cm–30cm of water by the same apparatus described for fixation of lung (Ludwig, 1979b). The canula is inserted into the cardia and the pylorus is clamped. After fixation has been completed, the luminal surface should be exposed. In the monogastric stomach, this

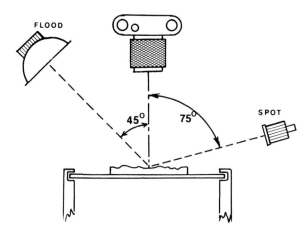

Figure 4.7. Texture light (spotlight) plus flood fill-in lamp. Courtesy of *Journal of Animal Science.*

should be done by cutting along both the lesser and greater curvatures. If necessary, color can be restored. However, photographs of fresh gastric mucosa are superior.

Intestines

Displacement, torsion, intussusception, and infarctions are best photographed *in situ.* In large animals it may be necessary to take two photographs, a "long shot" for orientation and a "close-up" to reveal details. The challenge is to obtain both of these in one photograph, but this can usually be done only in small animals. The gastrointestinal tracts of small laboratory animals are short and can be laid in one piece in either horizontal or vertical loops, with the stomach at the top left. The intestine is opened with an enterotome along its antimesenteric border. This procedure is facilitated if the mesentery is cut as closely as possible to the intestine as it is removed from the abdomen so that the gut can lie straight. However, photography of intestines has the same difficulties as described previously for the esophagus, that is, to "fill the frame" and yet show sufficient length of the gut. Options include horizontal rows (Fig. 4.8), vertical rows (Fig. 4.9), a single row, or an isolated loop with its mesentery to the top of the frame (Fig. 4.10).

Individual horizontal strips of gut are to be preferred to a continuous strip curved into rows. If vertical strips are used, the cranial ends of the intestine should be at the top of the frame. Pieces should be of uniform size with neatly cut edges. Irregularly sized pieces of gut with ragged

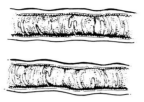

Figure 4.8.

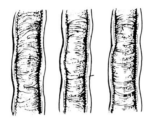

Figure 4.9.

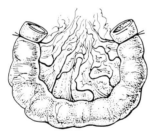

Figure 4.10.

edges are distracting. One of the greatest challenges is "proportioning," that is choosing the ratio between the sizes of the specimen and background. To minimize background, the strips of gut should be reasonably close together but separated by a distance equal to about two-thirds of the width of the opened gut. The background visible at the top and bottom of the box should be half the width of the opened gut. This makes for pleasant proportioning. Leaving a wide space between pieces means that the center of the field and thus the center of interest is empty.

A photograph of an intact loop of intestine with its mesentery (Fig. 4.10) and lymph nodes (in those species with mesenteric lymph nodes close to the gut, e.g. ruminant) can be very informative. Swollen lymph nodes and lymphangitis, as occur in Johne's disease (Mouwen and deGroot, 1982) are made more visible by the use of a dark or black background. Swollen lymph nodes can be incised and sequential photographs can be taken as the loop of intestine is opened along either its antimesenteric or lateral border to expose the contents (e.g. fibrinous casts in salmonellosis).

Depiction of the mucosa requires texture lighting. Vertical or horizontal formats are both suitable, depending on the direction of the folds in the wall of the intestine. With the specimen illuminated by one low-placed texture light, we rotate the background and specimen to find the point at which modeling is suitable and specular highlights are minimal. Then the camera is repositioned to frame the specimen correctly. Unfortunately, specular highlights can be quite numerous. These are increased even more if the specimen is washed with water or Jores' solution. Intestinal contents should be removed gently by a spatula, without washing, if possible. Also, besides producing specular highlights, washing the mucosa of the gastrointestinal tract detaches superficial epithelial cells, thus producing a less than optimal histological specimen. Therefore, if specimens are to be fixed optimally, neutral buffered 10% formalin (NBF) should be used to wash off ingesta and debris. This formalin wash causes the tunica muscularis to contract and pucker and partially degrades colors, and such specimens are not optimal for photography. If both optimal fixation and photography of gut are required, representative areas should be taken for each purpose. Diverticula can be demonstrated best by distending the isolated segment of gut with either 10% NBF or air. Air distended gut is dried in a stream of warm air. Intraluminal growths can be fixed in the unopened gut by the same technique described above for stomach (Ludwig, 1979b).

Liver

Anatomical displacement of the liver, such as through a diaphragmatic hernia, and alterations in size are best photographed with the liver *in situ.* Additional photographs may be made after the liver has been removed from the body and carefully dissected free of the diaphragm and attached ligaments. The best procedure for preparing the liver for photography is for it to need no special preparation. If the liver can be removed without contamination and thus requires no blotting, rinsing or sponging, it will photograph without excess specular highlights and with a "bloom" on its surface. Water should not come in contact with the liver's surface, as drops of water cause grey spots. Jores' solution lightens the blue-red color of the normal liver to bright red and increases the reflectivity of the serosa, resulting in the production of numerous specular highlights. If photography is delayed, particularly if the relative humidity of the room is low, the liver capsule is likely to dry, crinkle and become opaque. To prevent this, necropsy and specimen photography rooms should be humidified and maintained at a temperature of 68°F to 70°F. Exposure to studio lights should be minimized and framing and focusing of the specimen should be carried out using diffuse, low-level room lighting. Studio lights should be turned on only briefly to check modeling, position of shadows and specular highlights.

If similar lesions are present on both the visceral and parietal surfaces, the visceral surface is usually the more suitable for photography because:

1. It's surface is flatter and this causes fewer specular highlights, which are a problem on the parietal surface because of its curvature.
2. The flatter surface requires less depth of field, which is a significant advantage with the livers of very small animals.
3. The gallbladder (absent in the horse and rat) is visible and helps orient the viewer.

Because of its size and curved shape, the liver will usually have to be illuminated by two lights to avoid shadows. However, where surface texture is important such as in a cirrhotic liver, a main light or a main light with reduced fill-in illumination will be required. Photographs should be made of the whole organ and also close-ups of individual lesions such as nodules on the cirrhotic liver or focal granulomas in salmonellosis.

The cut surface of a liver can reveal characteristic lesions such as the nutmeg liver of chronic passive congestion. The most important requirement for successful preparation of liver slices is to cut uniformly thick pieces without any serrations. A sharp-bladed knife, sufficiently long to cut through the liver completely in one slice, is required. Ludwig (1979b) uses a custom-made knife, 30 inches long and 1 inch high for cutting human livers. An 18-inch straight knife is available commercially (No. 715 Post Mortem Knife, Lipshaw Manufacturing Co., Detroit, Michigan) and is sufficiently long to cut the livers of many of the smaller animals. The cut surface may or may not require delicate blotting, but blotting should be avoided if possible. The surface should be illuminated by one light to reduce specular highlights. If highlights are objectionable, then the procedures recommended above for their reduction (i.e. using left and right lights independently and rotating the specimen) should be tried. If the liver slice is not of uniform thickness, a portion of it may be in shadow or the depth of field may be inadequate. The background should be tilted slightly to bring the surface of the liver parallel with the film plane.

Sometimes a slice of liver will have a ragged surface, particularly if the cut is through a fragile necrotic mass or tumor. These specimens not only look unattractive but also the fine projections of the ragged edge may reflect numerous specular highlights. If the appearance of the specimen cannot be improved by trimming and specular highlights cannot be reduced by using one light or rotating the specimen, then the method of Gibson (1949) should be tried. He recommended immersion in physiological saline, pressing the jagged surface relatively flat with a glass plate and illuminating the specimen by two lamps at 45° lighting angles. Other precautions for immersion photography are described under "Specular Highlights." Multiple slices in a photograph should be avoided (Halsman and Ishak, 1977) as they merely divide the viewer's interest.

The dorsal border of the slice should be oriented towards the top of the frame. Livers of some species are frequently incorrectly oriented in photographs. The livers of carnivores and pigs have their long dimensions approximately transversely in the body (Shummer et al., 1979) and thus are correctly oriented in a horizontal format (Fig. 4.11). However, ruminants have the longer dimension approximately dorso-ventral and their livers should be photographed in a vertical format (Fig. 4.12). The long dimension of the horse's liver *in situ* is oblique from right-dorsal to left-ventral. To be absolutely correct, the liver should be placed obliquely in a horizontal format, but a liver arranged with its long dimension horizontally in a photograph is acceptable.

Pancreas

Photographs of pancreases are taken to show changes in size due to atrophy, nodular hyperplasia, neoplasia, or inflammation and blockage of excretory ducts and the adjacent bile duct by neoplasia. Changes in size are not easy to appreciate in a photograph of an isolated pancreas. In our necropsy technique for carnivores, the stomach, duodenum, pancreas and liver are removed in one block to allow dissection of ducts and examination of their relationships. Smaller than normal pancreases due to hypoplasia or atrophy can be appreciated if the stomach, duodenum,

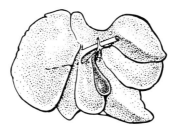

Figure 4.11. Correct anatomic orientation of carnivore and porcine livers.

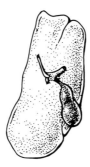

Figure 4.12. Correct anatomic orientation of ruminant livers. This requires a vertical camera format.

pancreas and mesoduodenum are photographed in one field with the mesentery stretched to show the pancreas. The same type of preparation can be used for cases of pancreatitis, although these should be photographed *in situ* first, to show any adjacent peritonitis or fat necrosis. If neoplasia involves the (common) bile duct, then the liver, stomach, duodenum and pancreas should be included in the one field for orientation, and fine detail shown in other close-up photographs of the neoplasm and ducts.

Circulatory System

Blood Vessels

As part of anatomical studies, photographs are frequently made to illustrate the location of arteries and veins. DelCampo (1974) described a technique of clearing (rendering transparent) tissues after the vessels had been injected with red or blue latex or gelatin dyed with either India ink, carmine red or Berlin blue. The cleared specimen was transilluminated and photographed.

In pathology, the most frequent vascular lesions are thrombi and emboli. Arterial and venous thrombi should be photographed *in situ* with the vessel opened, and later after removal from the body. *In situ* photographs are far more informative because they reveal location. If thrombi in the pulmonary artery are revealed during dissection of the heart, the pulmonary artery should be opened into the lung parenchyma. "Saddle" thrombi at the bifurcation of the aorta are more visible and their position easier to appreciate if, after removal of the abdominal viscera, the aorta and iliac arteries are opened *in situ* along their ventral midlines. The body should be oriented vertically in the photograph, and modeling lighting should be used either without fill-in illumination or with reduced fill-in illumination. Close-up photographs of vessels *in situ* may not be completely successful because of inadequate depth of field. Blood vessels are usually not in one plane and may extend beyond the available depth of field and thus be out of focus. To overcome this difficulty, the aorta and iliac arteries should be dissected free, laid on a photographic background and rephotographed to reveal fine detail.

Mural thrombi in the celiac and cranial mesenteric arteries of equidae, secondary to verminous arteritis, are difficult to photograph *in situ.* One solution is to dissect free several centimeters of the caudal thoracic aorta and most of the abdominal aorta, along with the attached celiac and cranial mesenteric arteries and several centimeters of their branches (Fig. 4.13). To reveal the verminous arteritis, the usual dissection procedure is to open these vessels along their left lateral walls, because the body is necropsied, lying on its right side.

Figure 4.13.

Jugular veins thrombosed by trauma from multiple intravenous injections should be dissected in a similar manner. Photographs of the veins *in situ* will reveal the perivascular edema and hemorrhage. Another approach is to remove a portion of the vein intact and then slice it transversely to reveal the characteristicly laminated thrombus. If the thrombus is very friable, the vein and thrombus should be fixed first. Then the thrombus can be exposed either by transverse serial slices or through a window cut in the vessel wall (Lie, 1979). In photographing a trailing thrombus in an opened vessel, the conical end of the thrombus should be included so that the viewer can recognize the type of thrombus involved. If desired, color can be restored to fixed specimens. The extent and location of atheromatous or other changes in the walls of vessels can be clearly depicted by removing the vessel and slicing it into uniformly wide pieces. These are then stood on end in the vessel's anatomic position (Fig. 4.14). If the contralateral vessel is normal, it can be sliced similarly and used as a control to emphasize the differences.

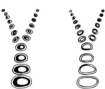

Figure 4.14. The vessels are cut into cross sections which are stood on end in the outline of the vessel and its branches, e.g. common carotid and internal and external carotid arteries. This allows the viewer to correlate the location of lesions with the segment of the vessel affected.

Photography of thrombi requires texture lighting, usually by one texture light alone or with a small amount of fill-in illumination. To obtain optimal modeling or texture under a standardized lighting system, the specimen and its background are rotated through approximately 30° clockwise and counter-clockwise to determine the best lighting angle. The intimal lesions in such chronic arteritides as equine verminous arteritis (in the cranial mesenteric and celiac arteries) and canine pulmonary arteritis due to Dirofilaria require texture lighting to reveal the proliferative nature of the lesions.

True aneurysms are relatively rare in veterinary medicine. These should be photographed *in situ,* if possible, and then fixed by perfusion. The artery should be removed and serially sliced transversely. Sections are placed in a vertical row, with the most cranial or dorsal towards the top of the frame. Color can be restored if required.

Pericardium

In some species of animals it is extremely easy to incise the pericardium accidentally during removal of the thoracic viscera. Thus, photographs to show distention of the pericardial sac by fluids are best made

with the heart *in situ.* Distended pericardial sacs should be photographed
unopened to show the shape and size and then opened on their mid-
lateral surface to show the nature of the contents. Allis forceps may be
used to hold the edges of the sac so that the contents do not escape. The
inflammatory response characteristic of acute pericarditis is a fibrinous
exudate followed by a fibrinopurulent exudate which may lead to replacement by granulation tissue resulting in an adhesive pericarditis. The
photographic challenge is to record the texture of these exudates on
parietal and visceral layers of the pericardium. Normal necropsy technique is to leave the heart attached to the lungs until the great vessels
have been opened. The opened pericardium can still be photographed
before detachment of the heart from the lungs. The pericardium should
be incised from apex to base and reflected to reveal any inflammatory
changes on the surface of both visceral and parietal layers. Because fibrin
loses its fibrillar appearance within five to ten minutes of exposure to air,
particularly if the temperature is high or the humidity is low, photographs should be taken immediately. The heart should be oriented
approximately vertically (Fig. 4.15), never horizontally, although its true
anatomic position is slightly oblique. A modeling light plus a fill-in
light will be needed to reveal the nature of the exudate and to illuminate
both sides of the heart. Later, the heart can be detached from the lungs
and rephotographed. Once the exudate has organized to granulation
tissue, removal of the pericardium may be impossible because of adhesions.
However, strands of granulation and fibrous tissue will be revealed on
incision of the parietal pericardium. The thickness of the granulation
tissue on the epicardium and the associated compensatory myocardial
hypertrophy in chronic cases are beautifully revealed by serial transverse slices through pericardium and heart. The thickness of these slices,
from 0.5cm to 2cm, will depend on the size of the heart.

Heart

As already described under "Pericardium," the heart should be oriented
vertically in photographs (Fig. 4.15). A vertical camera format is required
for the unopened heart and a horizontal one for the heart incised to
reveal the interior of the chambers. Photographs of the exterior of the
heart are taken to reveal changes in shape such as rounding or bifurcation of the apex due to cardiac failure. Thus, to emphasize the change in
outline, there should be good tonal contrast between the mahogany-
colored heart and the background. A light to mid-grey background is

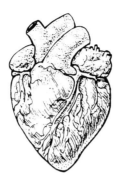

Figure 4.15.

suitable. Myocardial necrosis is relatively rare in veterinary medicine. However, pale necrotic foci, either infarcts or myodegeneration due, for example, to vitamin E/selenium deficiency will be more visible against a dark grey background.

Olsen (1973) states that "there is no standard method of opening the heart in human pathology and a variety of techniques have been described." In veterinary pathology the most frequently used method is to open the heart in the direction of blood flow, a method commonly ascribed to Virchow. However, the original Virchow method temporarily preserved the atrio-ventricular rings (Reiner, 1968), an advantage when evaluating the competence of valves. For example, a congenitally incompetent mitral valve can be viewed and photographed from the atrial side after a Virchow-style incision into the atrium. The wall of the dilated atrium is easily positioned by gloved hands to reveal the dilated atrio-ventricular orifice. Precautions in technique include not handling the valve cusps and not cutting through the valve commissures or the chordae tendineae (Olsen, 1973). An alternative method of dissection of the heart is to make serial transverse cuts across the ventricles. This method reveals ventricular hypertrophy dramatically and also shows the extent of myocardial necrosis caused by either infarction or nutritional myodegeneration. A similar transverse cut across the atria just dorsal to the atrio-ventricular valves has been used to expose these valves and allow their competency or stenosis to be demonstrated. Ventricles are filled with water, aortic and pulmonary arteries clamped, and the heart squeezed by a gloved hand to check for regurgitation through the atrio-ventricular valves.

Photographs of endocardium and heart valves are easy to obtain in hearts dissected by the Virchow method. Although many hearts have relatively flabby walls which can be folded back easily to expose the valves, hypertrophied hearts may have turgid walls and need retractors to expose the valves. The problem of retractors has been discussed (see "Retractors"). Generally, hands covered by clean well-fitting latex surgeon's gloves are less objectionable in photographs than makeshift wood or glass retractors or sutures fastened through the heart wall to pins on a frame outside of the photograph.

The most successful pictures of endocardium and valves are those taken immediately after death. Even in a small cadaver, such as that of a dog, held for 12 hours in a cold room at 4°C, the endocardium will loose its "bloom" and, after washing with water, will assume a dull grey appearance. In these cases it is wiser to attempt to remove blood and clots by wiping with sponges rather than by washing with water. After taking photographs, the endocardium can be washed with physiological saline in the hope that it will appear better than in the first photographs. To record the texture of the heart valves and the modeling of the interior of the ventricles, a modeling light with either no or reduced fill-in illumination is required.

Endocrine System

Because endocrine organs are extremely small, most photographs are taken to show changes in size. Examples are goiter in lambs and birds, pituitary chromophobe adenomas in rats, hyperplastic parathyroids in renal failure, atrophy of the adrenal cortex secondary to prolonged steroid administration and nodular cortical hyperplasia of the adrenals. Thus, the major decision is how best to demonstrate changes in size. Such changes can be appreciated only if an endocrine organ can be compared with an adjacent organ or its companion if it is paired. *Pituitary* enlargements due to neoplasms or cysts are more obvious if the pituitary is still attached to the brain, as, for example, a rat with a chromophobe adenoma. However, if the pituitary tumor has grown slowly, there may be little hint of its size until it has been removed. Only then will the cavity formed by compression of the brain be obvious. Enlarged parathyroid glands should be photographed attached to the thyroid gland in those species which have that anatomical arrangement. With careful dissection, both parathyroids and thyroids can be exposed *in situ* on the trachea in carnivores or on the common carotid arteries close to the thoracic inlet in birds. Congenital goiter in lambs may be visible through the skin as a gentle swelling from enlarged thyroids. Revealing these in photographs will require modeling light to emphasize their shape. After the skin has been reflected, the bilaterally enlarged thyroids should be photographed *in situ* from a ventral viewpoint. Following the removal of the thoracic and neck organs *en bloc,* the thyroids should be readily visible in a dorsal view, usually after minimal blunt dissection. This block of organs should be positioned vertically and a vertical camera format used.

Goiter in birds can also be dramatic. Avian thyroids are located near the thoracic inlet and the bird should be placed in a vertical orientation and illuminated by a modeling light. Framing is very important, as it is necessary to orient the viewer and at the same time direct attention to the enlarged thyroids. To do this, usually the head, neck and some thorax should be included. A second close-up photograph of the lower neck and upper thorax can be taken to record the enlarged thyroids in greater detail.

Nodular hyperplasia of the *adrenal cortex* should be photographed in the intact adrenal, or otherwise in cross sections. Adrenal infarcts and cortical hemorrhages, frequently seen in horses with toxemia, are visible only on the cut surfaces. Transverse slices should be of a uniform width so that when placed on end, their upper surfaces will be in the same plane. This is necessary because of the shallow depth of field at RR's approaching 1:1. For orientation purposes, the convention of left gland to the left side of the frame and cranial pole to the top should be observed. Modeling or texture lighting will be required.

Neoplasms of the adrenal infiltrating into the caudal vena cava should be photographed *in situ* and then the block of kidneys, renal vessels, aorta and caudal vena cava removed and rephotographed before and after the vessels are opened. Usually, a ventral view will be used and thus the right kidney and adrenal will be on the left side of the frame, but their cranial poles should be towards the top of the frame. A horizontal format will be required to frame both kidneys and adrenals.

Lympho-Reticular System

Organs of this system which may be photographed include lymph nodes, spleen, thymus and lymphatics. Photographs of these organs can be unsatisfactory unless the pathologist first decides what feature he really wants to record. Photographs of lymph nodes are usually intended to show:

1. **Changes in Size.** Lymph nodes are widely scattered over the body. If a generalized lymphadenopathy is to be shown, the dissection will have to be planned so that enlarged superficial lymph nodes are revealed. The usual necropsy procedure is to reflect the uppermost legs dorsally in a cadaver in lateral recumbency. However, in this case, the best procedure is to leave the legs in their normal position and the body in lateral recumbency and remove the skin and excess fat to reveal the superficial lymph nodes such as the mandibular, prescapular (caudal superficial cervical) and prefemoral. If the lymph nodes are very large and the body is cachectic, swelling of the lymph nodes will be visible through the skin. They can be photographed with suitable modeling lighting to emphasize the swollen lymph nodes. Lighting is more pleasant if the cadaver faces into the main (modeling) light, as this prevents a shadow falling in front of the face. Either full or reduced fill-in illumination will be needed to illuminate the shadows, otherwise these will have little or no detail.

2. **Location of Affected Lymph Nodes.** For example, metastases in the tracheobronchial lymph nodes from pulmonary adenocarcinoma.

3. **Shape and Texture of Surfaces.**
   a. outer surfaces to show changes in shape such as nodules from metastasis or abscesses.
   b. cut surfaces to illustrate either diffuse or focal changes. Diffuse changes include obliteration of normal architecture from neoplasia such as malignant lymphoma and edema and reddening from acute inflammation. Focal lesions include metastases, focal granulomas and abscesses.

4. **Color.** Tracheobronchial lymph nodes in advanced pulmonary anthracosis are black. Regional lymph nodes draining a hemorrhagic site may be red from hemorrhage or brown from hemosiderin. Lymph nodes with metastatic malignant melanoma may be black.

Thus, the dissection method to display these features best should be considered before the necropsy proceeds. Regional lymph nodes may not be visible until fat or serosa, such as the mediastinal pleura over the tracheobronchial lymph nodes, has been dissected away. Isolated lymph nodes should be removed intact and dissected free of fat and connective tissue without nicks or cuts. This can be done easily by a knife held vertically next to the lymph node. As the knife is moved back and forth gently, the fat and fascia are pulled under the knife, with forceps held in the prosector's other hand. The procedure is quick and efficient. It is also easier to remove adventitia from a lymph node before it is sectioned transversely. Views of the exterior of lymph nodes are usually uninformative unless there are significant changes in size, shape or color. To avoid serrations on the cut surface, transverse sectioning of a lymph node to reveal cortex and medulla should be made with a single stroke of a long-bladed knife. So that slices are uniformly wide, the cut should be made without undue pressure.

The cut surface should be photographed immediately before drying changes the texture of the surface. It is essential that the freshly cut surface not be blotted or washed, as these procedures will change texture and increase specular highlights. As the objective of photographing cut surfaces is to record surface texture (e.g. smooth and grey with malignant lymphoma, edematous in acute lymphadenitis and caseous in tuberculosis), illumination by one low-placed texture light is required. If the slice or slices are not uniformly thick, some portion of them may be in shadow. Such slices should be propped up with modeling clay or alternatively the background tilted a little. Convention is to orient slices so the hilus is towards the bottom of the frame. This is aesthetically pleasing because drainage is from the cortex at the top to the efferent lymphatics at the bottom of the frame. Sometimes one cross section is sufficient; sometimes two or more are needed to show variation in the lesion. However, the more cross sections in the photograph, the more the viewer's attention is divided. Thus, a minimum number of cross sections should be included.

Lymphatics

Normal lymphatics are rarely visible. The exceptions are lymphatics of the mesentery distended with white chyle after a fatty meal. Lymphatics dilated by an inflammatory exudate draining from an inflamed area or by ectasia may also be visible. Lymphatics are usually transparent and thus are more visible viewed against a dark background. Mesenteric lymphatics filled with chyle or affected with lymphangitis as in Johne's disease are dramatically visible if the mesentery is spread over a black background. The usual necropsy procedure of freeing intestines by cutting them close to their mesenteric attachment is inappropriate in these cases. Therefore, if mesenteric lymph nodes are to be demonstrated, a loop of intestine and its mesentery should be removed *in toto* by cutting the root of the mesentery and transecting the intestines after double ligation of each end. Intestine and mesentery can then be spread over a black background to demonstrate the lymphatics in the mesentery (Fig. 4.10).

Modeling or texture lighting with reduced or no fill-in illumination should be tried. Ectatic lymphatics are usually tortuous and distended with clear fluid. If they project above the surface of an organ such as the heart, they can be made more visible by illumination from a texture light.

Thymus

Photographs of thymus are used to record presence in older animals, location, size and tumors. Location and size as, for example, of the cervical portion of the bovine thymus, are best depicted *in situ*, as any appreciation of location is lost after removal. Photographs of tumors of the mediastinal thymus *in situ* usually show no more than enlargement. This enlargement may be more obvious after removal of thoracic organs from the body. Another alternative is to place the body in lateral recumbency, remove the upper thoracic wall and upper lung and photograph the mediastinum *in situ*. Modeling lighting will be required to reveal the size and shape of the mediastinal mass, but as this will cast deep shadows, fill-in illumination (from a 45° light) will be required. However, in the standardized position, both lights are of equal intensity and the fill-in illumination will be excessive and eliminate the shadows from the modeling light. Reduced fill-in illumination should be tried and the effect on the modeling of the contours of the mediastinal mass checked in the viewfinder.

Spleen

Photographs of the spleen are frequently taken to show size, emphasizing Smith and Jones' (1957) observation that spleens come in two sizes: "too large and too small." Because of variations in body size of different animals, photographs of isolated spleens rarely succeed in dramatizing changes in size, unless a normal control is included. Alternatively the spleen can be photographed *in situ* where comparison with other abdominal organs is possible. If splenomegaly is to be depicted photographically, a departure from standard necropsy procedure may be required. Most domestic animals, except horses, are necropsied lying on their left sides and thus their spleens are either not visible or only partly visible when the right abdominal wall is removed. A far more dramatic photograph can be made if the abdomen is opened from the left side.

For optimal preparation, the spleen should not be congested. Therefore, barbiturates and chloral hydrate should not be used for anesthesia or euthanasia, as they induce splenomegaly from congestion in the storage- or semi-storage-type spleens present in most domestic animals. Another common cause of splenomegaly is neoplasms. The commonest primary splenic neoplasms in the dog are hemangioma and hemangiosarcoma. These splenic neoplasms are often difficult to photograph, because they are very dark red or sometimes bluish-red from the blood in their vascular sinuses. There is a tendency to underexpose, with the result that photographs have little detail in the very dark areas. A major problem is the prolonged oozing of blood from the cut surface. There are several alternative techniques to control oozing. The best procedure is prevention at euthanasia by rapid exsanguination under deep non-barbiturate anesthesia. If the spleen is congested at necropsy, the splenic pedicle can be clamped and severed. The spleen, covered with a saline-soaked gauze to prevent drying, should be placed in a refrigerator overnight, in the hope that much of the blood will clot. Immersion fixation of whole spleens is unsatisfactory, as both the large size and the thick capsule retard penetration of fixative. Also, perfusion fixation may not be successful unless the blood is washed out first (Ludwig, 1979b). Alternatively, the spleen can be cut in cross sections (for example, across a hemangioma and adjacent normal splenic tissue) and held in Jores' solution for several days until oozing ceases. The Jores' solution will have to be replaced several times. The final result will be a cross section of a spleen with falsified red colors but with excellent rendition of the texture of the tumor and spleen. Another alternative is to fix a slice of spleen in Schein's fixative and restore the color by the hydrosulfite technique.

Hyperplastic nodules and metastatic neoplasms such as squamous cell carcinomas or mast cell tumors are usually quite discrete, and lesions should be incised sufficiently to reveal their texture. The canine spleen should be photographed in a vertical format (Fig. 4.16), because this approximates to its anatomic position. This position also gives better modeling under the standardized lights than if the spleen were arranged with its longitudinal axis horizontal. To show the color and texture of a nodule on the spleen, it should be incised in a direction that allows the cut surface to be illuminated by the main (modeling) light. Fill-in lighting may be needed to illuminate shadows.

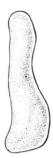

Figure 4.16.

For monochrome photography of lesions in a congested spleen, transverse sections (0.5cm to 2cm thick) of spleen with lesions should be placed in Jores' solution, as described above for color photography, or in 10% NBF or Shein's fixative for several days to a week depending on the thickness of the slice. Later, these pieces can be photographed to show the contour of the nodule and then cut in cross sections to reveal the surface texture of the normal and adjacent neoplastic tissues. If the texture is adequately revealed, there will be no need to resort to color restoration. However, if contrast is low, color can be restored to Schein's fixed material by hydrosulfite (see "Color Restoration"). If fixation has been in 10% formalin for a long period, Meiller's technique is the method of choice for restoration of color.

Muscular System

Muscles in Situ

Photographs of muscles *in situ* are only successful if there is some striking alteration in color or size, for example, from denervation atrophy or muscular hypertrophy. Muscles may be discolored green in eosinophilic myositis, red from hemorrhage in myorrhexis and pale grey from necrosis, calcification, lipomatosis or in malignant hyperthermia of pigs. Symmetrical differences in adjacent muscles, as for example those caused by malignant hyperthermia in porcine lumbar muscles, are best demonstrated in a transverse slice through lumbar muscles and vertebrae. Sequential dissection and photography is the best way to proceed. Muscles should be dissected free without knife cuts or nicks and the fascia removed to reveal the muscle itself. Muscles which are very dark from congestion or hemorrhage are extremely difficult to photograph.

Circumscribed lesions which contrast with adjacent normal muscles (e.g. calicified Trichinella) photograph well. This is particularly true of muscles of large animals photographed *in situ* with electronic flash.

Isolated Muscles

Photographs of isolated muscles are taken to record changes in color (see above) or changes in texture such as amorphous necrotic areas or edematous or gas-filled areas in Clostridial myositis. These changes are best appreciated if the specimen includes both normal and abnormal areas. A desirable procedure is to dissect the whole muscle free and slice it in the direction of its fibers. This is not possible in pennate or semi-pennate muscles or in muscles with fibers running in various directions (e.g. temporalis). A uniformly wide slice should be cut through the normal muscle and lesion with one cut of a straight long-bladed knife so that no serrations from to-and-fro cuts are produced. Because most muscles, particularly those of the limbs, have their long axis running dorso-ventrally, fibers should be oriented to run vertically in the photograph. Fortunately, this is often the optimal orientation for lighting, with the modeling or texture light coming from the top left. A major problem is specular highlights reflected from cut surfaces, particularly if edema or exudate is present. Also, specular highlights reflect from each individual muscle fasciculus and can be troublesome even if only one light is used. Polarization may be necessary. Specular highlights are particularly plentiful on those muscles which will not lie flat (e.g. diaphragm). If specular highlights cannot be controlled by repositioning the specimen in relation to the lights or by the use of polarized light, the only alternative may be to fix the muscle and photograph it under fluid (e.g. in a Kennedy tank). This will allow the pale necrotic and fibrous areas to be seen clearly (see "Specular Highlights"). Although most lesions are best demonstrated by slicing the muscle in the direction of its fibers, the gas bubbles of clostridial myositis are more dramatically presented in transverse slices which clearly show the separation of fibers by gas.

Unilateral lesions such as hypertrophy, atrophy or fibrosis can be demonstrated more strikingly by including both left and right muscles in the one frame, the normal one being used as a control. Photographs of focal or segmental necrosis, abscesses, parasitic granulomas, calcification, discolorations due to injected medicaments, eosinophilic myositis and localized areas of gas gangrene, which are all lesions with good color contrast between affected and normal areas, photograph well. For these, a modeling light with full or reduced fill-in illumination is required.

Nervous System

Brain

In veterinary pathology, it is usual to disarticulate the head before removing the calvaria to expose the brain. At that time, lesions such as cerebellar hypoplasia or cerebellar coning with the vermis protruding through the foramen magnum may be visible. Photographs of these lesions may be more dramatic at this stage of dissection than after the calvaria has been removed. Neoplasms such as meningiomas on the dorsal surface of the parietal cortex should be photographed after the removal of the calvaria but before removal of the brain from the skull, as removal may result in displacement of the tumor. Unfortunately, these types of photographs are difficult to take, mainly because of the difficulties in positioning the head and setting up desirable lighting. If the head is positioned on its ventral surface after removal of the mandible and calvaria, the plane of the brain's surface slopes steeply from the surface of the parietal lobes to the medulla and this distance is usually beyond the depth of field for the RR required to fill the frame. Also, the angle of view is not really suitable. The problem of positioning the brain can be overcome if the horizontal arm of the camera stand can be rotated on its horizontal axis so that the camera len's optical axis is at right angles to the plane from the top of the parietal cortex to the medulla. Unfortunately, relatively few stands have this feature. Positioning of the head for dorso-lateral or caudal views is extremely difficult. The simplest procedure is to press the skull into a ball of modeling clay to see if it will hold fast. Another technique is to saw the skull transversely across the nasal bones and stand the head on this surface, thus positioning the caudal surface of the brain towards the camera. The technique works well for most small short skulls. We have used this technique to position a feline head with cerebellar coning of the vermis through the foramen magnum. If neither of these methods will position the skull correctly, another alternative is to hold the head with hands covered by scrupulously clean surgeon's gloves, preferably with the hands placed as inconspicuously as possible. To overcome movement, exposure should be short or made by electronic flash.

After the examination of the exterior of the brain, the usual procedure is to fix it completely before photography, because the fresh brain tends to distort under its own weight as it sits on the background. However, purulent meningitis, visible brain abscesses and metastatic tumors should be photographed while the brain is fresh and color is retained. Usually, dissection of the fresh brain is to be avoided, because cutting the soft brain results in distortion and uniformly thin slices cannot be obtained. If dissection before fixation is absolutely essential (e.g. to cut to expose an abscess for culture or to obtain material for histological study), the brain can be made firmer by refrigeration at 4°C for 30 minutes (Okazaki and Campbell, 1979). These authors also recommend that dissection of the unfixed (human) brain be limited to no more than 3 to 4 coronal cuts. In brains with symmetrical or disseminated infections, the brain can be bisected midsagittally and one-half used for histological examination and the other for microbiological or chemical examinations. Unfortunately, slices of half the brain are not photogenic and we avoid midsagittal bisection if photography is important.

The shape of the brain can be retained by fixing it in 10% NBF to which just sufficient 37% formaldehyde solution (full-strength commercial formalin) has been added to cause the brain to float. Floating prevents the flattening that occurs when the brain lies on the bottom of a container. An alternative method is to suspend the brain in fixative by a string around the circle of Willis. Okazaki and Campbell (1979) advise against incising the corpus callosum which is sometimes recommended in the hope of allowing fixative into the lateral ventricles. Such a technique certainly can cause separation of the cerebral hemispheres and distortion of the brain slices. Fixation should continue for at least 48 to 72 hours for small brains (e.g. canine), 4 to 5 days for bovine and equine and 1 to 2 weeks for larger brains (e.g. human). The period of fixation should be sufficiently long to render the brain firm and amenable to slicing but still retain some of the natural color on the cut surface. If the specimen is particularly bloody, the formalin should be replaced after 12 to 24 hours to prevent undesirable discoloration of the specimen (Okazaki and Campbell, 1979), a defect which is particularly obvious in fixed grey brain slices. After fixation, gyri and sulci do not collapse, and alterations in their shapes can be photographed easily with texture lighting. If the dorsal or ventral surfaces of the whole brain are to be photographed, the

brain should be oriented with its long axis vertical (Figs. 4.17 and 4.18).
For lateral views, the brain should be positioned with its long axis
horizontal (Fig. 4.19). Inclusion of a normal control for comparison will
emphasize differences in size (e.g. cerebellar hypoplasia). Both brains
should be vertical and positioned side by side for dorsal or ventral views
and one above the other in lateral views. Modeling lighting with full or
occasionally reduced fill-in illumination is required.

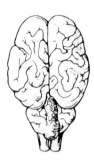 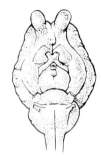 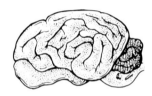

Figure 4.17. (*Left*) Dorsal and Fig. 4.18 (*Center*) ventral surfaces of the brain should be
viewed with the brain positioned with its rostral pole to the top of the frame.
Figure 4.19. (*Right*) The brain may be positioned horizontally only when a lateral surface
(or medial surface of a hemisphere) is viewed.

The conventional method of examining brains is, after fixation, to
slice them transversely through well-recognized external landmarks (e.g.
optic chiasma, mamillary bodies, rostral colliculi, etc.). Thus, in small
animals slices may be 1mm to 5mm thick and in large animals 2mm to
20mm. Each slice should be uniformly thick and perfectly flat and free of
any knife marks. For large brains, a special brain knife should be used.
Its blade is 12 to 18 inches long, 1-½ inches high, straight, thin, flexible
and without a bevel. Disposable 18 inch long brain knives are available
(Feather Industries Ltd., Tokyo, Japan). The blade is moistened with
glycerine, physiological saline, water or 10% NBF "to prevent tissue
sticking and tearing" (Mallory and Wright, 1918). To avoid leaving knife
marks, the brain should be cut with one stroke of the knife, from heel to
toe and without undue pressure (La Bossiere, 1976). A razor blade is
better for cutting the small brains of laboratory animals. If the brain is
not firm, slices of uniform width can still be cut if the rostral surface of
the brain is pressed gently against a vertical glass or Plexiglas plate (Fig.

4.20). This holds the brain flat and the prosector can see if the whole of the rostral face is in contact with the plate. If the interior of the brain is not fixed uniformly, photography can be delayed 24 hours to allow uniform fixation. However, some lesions such as hemorrhagic infarcts or tumors such as astrocytomas should be photographed immediately to record the display of colors.

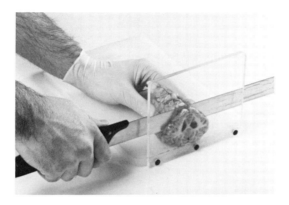

Figure 4.20. Apparatus to facilitate the cutting of uniformly thin brain slices. The cut surface of the brain is pressed gently against the Plexiglas plate until the whole surface of the brain is in contact. The base is a polyethylene cutting board.

The convention in human pathology is to display the brain slices with the right side of the slice to the right of the frame. This corresponds to a caudal view of the brain slices. They are arranged in two or more vertical rows, with the most rostral at the top left and the most caudal at the bottom right (Nickey, 1977; Okazaki and Campbell, 1979). Animals' brains are comparatively small and only one to two vertical rows will be needed. If it is necessary to record the extent or distribution of lesions throughout the whole brain (e.g. canine metastatic hemangiosarcoma), all slices should be photographed. However, the viewer's attention is more concentrated if only several well chosen slices are used to illustrate the *extent* of the lesions (Fig. 4.21). To depict the *characteristic* lesions, one slice alone should be photographed (Fig. 4.22). Ishak and Halsman (1977) point out that a single coronal section of the (human) brain, through a neoplasm or an area of encephalomalacia, may tell the whole story, whereas including all of the sections of brain, arranged like sausages, makes each individual section proportionately smaller and probably confuses and irritates the viewer. Inclusion of a normal (control) section is sometimes desirable if lesions are subtle (e.g. mild hypomyelinogenisis) or if it is wished to show the dramatic differences between the affected and normal (e.g. marked hydrocephalus). However, the control sections should always be subservient to the one with lesions. For this reason it is essential that the viewer's eye see the affected brain slice first and thus the control should be on the right if two sections are placed side by side in a horizontal format, or below if slices are placed in a vertical format. The viewer can be frustrated if no lesions are detected in the first specimen that the eye sees. To record fine detail, a portion of a slice can be photographed but the field of view should include sufficient landmarks, such as a lateral ventricle or corpus striatum, to allow the viewer to orient himself (Fig. 4.23).

Vertically arranged slices are suitable for monochrome prints, as they can be enlarged to the column width of a journal. Slices should not touch or overlap (Okazaki and Campbell, 1979), as later it may be necessary to choose only one slice in a photograph for publication. Slices are oriented by moving them until their midlines are over a vertical line in the graticule of the camera's viewfinder. Full frame horizontal format views of an individual slice can also be centered on the lines in the viewfinder. The use of a focusing screen with several vertical and horizontal lines such as the Nikon E screen (Fig. 1.10) facilitates this orientation.

Background. The most suitable background depends on whether the photograph is for a black-and-white print or a color transparency as well as on the features to be depicted. A clear white background is best for monochrome prints. This has been discussed under "Backgrounds". Black backgrounds are popular for photographs of brains and are particularly suitable if attention is to be directed to changes in outline such as asymmetry due to neoplasms, brain abscesses or cerebral cortical atrophy. However, if the attention of the viewer is to be directed to detail *within* the slice, a less dark background is indicated and a dark grey is the most suitable. Colored backgrounds and their distortion of color perception have been discussed under "Backgrounds." In cases where color is not important (e.g. in photographs of fixed brain slices to demonstrate anatomical landmarks), colored backgrounds have a psychological advantage. Brain slices on a sky blue background are reminiscent of clouds in a blue sky. This combination retains the viewer's attention for longer periods than dark grey or black backgrounds which are somber and depressing, particularly when large numbers of slides are shown.

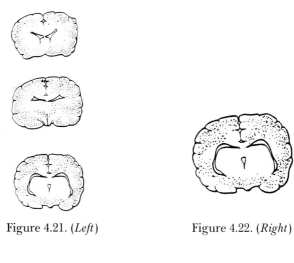

Figure 4.21. (*Left*)   Figure 4.22. (*Right*)

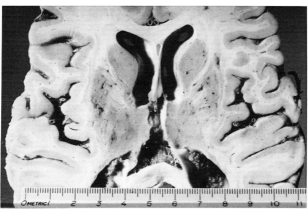

Figure 4.23. Human brain. Binswanger's disease. One texture light (see Fig. 3.5) was used to bring out the fine perivascular depressions. For publication, the ruler would be trimmed off and replaced by a 1cm scale marker.

Lighting. While brain slices are often considered to be textureless, in fact, sulci, small depressions, blood vessels, ventricles and changes in texture in the surface of lesions such as metastatic carcinomas appear in moderate relief when illuminated by one modeling or texture light (Fig. 4.23). Slices appear pale, featureless, ill-defined and uninteresting when illuminated by flat lighting, for example, from two lights at 45°. Necrotic areas stained by blood or which have advanced to the friable stage are readily visible with texture lighting and photograph well. Early malacic areas may not be detectable on visual examination, but Markson and

Wells (1982) have shown that when such areas in ruminant brains are illuminated by a UV light of a wavelength of 365 nm, they autofluoresce yellow and are readily visible. The area illuminated by the UV lamp may be only several centimeters in diameter. If a 55mm lens is used, its short working distance will mean that the UV lamp will illuminate the subject at an oblique angle and this may produce a small, unevenly illuminated field. The obvious solution is to use a longer focal length lens (e.g. 105mm on a 35mm camera) with the lamp positioned next to the lens's rim. The longer working distance of this lens allows the UV lamp to be moved closer to axial lighting (Fig. 3.3) and thus give more even illumination. Care must be taken to use a matte background which does not reflect the image of the lamp into the camera. Fluorescing lesions can be photographed in a darkroom on daylight film. Exposure has to be determined by trial and error. Also, different filters, e.g. UV, yellow (Wratten 15), may have to be used over the camera's lens to reduce the UV and blue light reaching the film.

Hydrocephalus. Special techniques are necessary to preserve the neonatal hydrocephalic brain. Even normal neonatal brains are soft and easily damaged and distorted. They should be fixed by floating them in 10% NBF by the addition of 37% formaldehyde solution, as described above. Fetal and neonatal brains have a high water content, and 20% formalin solutions have been recommended because 10% NBF may not harden sufficiently (Okazaki and Campbell, 1979). Hydrocephalic brains have thin cortices which collapse or are damaged or distorted easily during the removal of the calvaria (Laurence and Martin, 1959). To preserve their shape, these brains must be fixed *in situ* and this can be done by the injection of formalin into the lateral ventricles through the open fontanelles or through a burr hole in the calvaria, or by perfusion fixation of the brain *in situ* or both. Warm 10% formalin in 70% alcohol (Pangilinan, 1974) or even 15% formalin (Laurence and Martin, 1959) have been used. Emery and Marshall (1965) warned that if a large amount of fluid is withdrawn, the cerebral hemispheres and lateral ventricles will collapse and the brain will not retain its normal shape and position, thus defeating the object of fixing the brain *in situ*. They recommend that in children, a 10 ml syringe be used to remove no more than 10 ml of fluid and then replace it with 10ml of 37% formaldehyde (commercial formalin). The procedure should be repeated approximately 10 times in children. Because the brains of most animals are smaller than those of children, the number of injections should be adjusted to the size of the animal. Laurence and Martin (1959) described a technique for the preparation of a specimen to demonstrate hydrocephalus and hydromyelia *in situ* in the skull and vertebral column in a human. Fixation was by injection of 15% formalin into the lateral ventricles followed by perfusion fixation with 10% formalin via the carotid arteries and then immersion of the skull and vertebral column in 10% formalin for at least a week and preferably three weeks. The specimen was sawn midsagittally to reveal the cranial and vertebral lesions.

Dura Mater

Lesions in the dura mater are relatively infrequent in veterinary pathology. The dura may be discolored yellow by bilirubin in jaundice or green in sheep with the Dubin-Johnson syndrome. In young animals extra-dural hemorrhage may result in dissection of the dura from the periosteum. In this position, the hemorrhage will be visible as the skull is rongeured away, or will be seen between the dura and the periosteum on the isolated skull cap. The remainder of the cerebral dura may be examined after removal of the brain when the dura lining the base and sides of the cranial vault is visible. Photography of this dura is extremely difficult because the head is awkward to position, making illumination of the cranial fossa difficult. The head can be stood on its base with its long axis horizontal and with the foramen magnum towards the 45° modeling light. This will illuminate the rostral fossa. The caudal end of the skull will frequently have to be elevated by black wooden blocks. Even though two lamps are used, only one is effectively illuminating the interior of the cranial vault and thus exposure should be based on one lamp.

Subdural hematomas on the lateral walls formed by the frontal bones are difficult to position so that they are visible to the camera. One alternative is to saw the head midsagittally and lay one half on its lateral surface propped up so that the midsagittal plane is horizontal and thus parallel to the film plane. Then the lateral wall of the rostral fossa will be visible to the camera and can be illuminated by one of the lamps.

Spinal Cord

Only a relatively small percentage of spinal cord lesions are visible on gross examination. These include neoplasms, abscesses, granulomas and malacic foci. Display of lesions depends on the method used to expose the spinal cord, which is usually done either by a dorsal laminectomy or by a sagittal saw cut into the vertebral canal just lateral to the spinal cord. Removal of the lateral wall of the vertebral canal by a band saw requires considerable skill, and errors may result in mutilation of the cord. One approach is to remove 2mm to 3mm thick slices of bone until the vertebral canal is just penetrated and then to make the final exposure of the spinal cord by using bone forceps, rongeurs or a Stryker saw. However, this does not make a pretty dissection. The most suitable approach to remove the cord is dictated by the location of the lesion.

Lesions on the dorsal aspect of the cord may be visible after dorsal laminectomy, but compressive lesions originating ventrally, caused, for example, by vertebral abscesses, vertebral body fractures or prolapsed intervertebral discs, are best seen after removal of the lateral wall of the vertebral canal. Compression lesions and compressed cords can be photographed *in situ,* and, after removal of the cord, the actual lesion responsible for the compression can be rephotographed. When it is desirable to preserve both the dorsal laminae and the intervertebral articular surfaces, the cord can be removed by sawing through the vertebral bodies in a horizontal plane just dorsal to the ventral surface of the vertebral canal. This works well with large animals, because there are several millimeters of space between the cord and the ventral surface of the vertebral canal. Later, the vertebrae can be reassembled to evaluate changes in them. Exposure of the vertebral canal may reveal extradural lesions such as malignant lymphoma common in cattle, meningiomas, metastatic neoplasms, osteogenic sarcomas extending from adjacent vertebrae, extruded intervertebral disc material and also intervertebral abscesses. These should be photographed *in situ.*

Lighting. This must be designed to emphasize changes in outline, e.g. elevation of the ventral wall of the vertebral canal by a vertebral fracture and changes in texture. Examples of the latter are the smooth grey of malignant lymphoma or the yellow caseous exudate of a tuberculous abscess. Thus, texture or modeling lighting is essential. Usually, the cord *in situ* in the vertebrae is placed with its long axis horizontal and with the cranial end towards the modeling or texture light which shines along the length of the spinal cord. It is desirable to check illumination by left and right lights independently to see which is the more effective. Also, the background and specimen should be rotated a little around the camera's axis to see the effect of changes in placement of shadows. As the light has to shine down the length of the vertebral canal after removal of the cord, there is little latitude for much rotation. Correctly placed, this light produces excellent results which appear natural. Fill-in illumination may not be required.

After removal of the cord, the dura is incised in a middorsal sagittal plane to expose the cord. Because the spinal cord is long and thin, it does not lend itself to photography as a whole. This is rarely required, as most visible lesions are confined to several cord segments, and close-up photographs are suitable as they fill the frame. Many lesions in the spinal cord, particularly compression lesions, result in a change in cord shape and so isolated cords, or cross sections, are best photographed on a black background to emphasize the shape of the outline. In photographs of the dorsal or ventral surfaces of a spinal cord, a vertical format is anatomically correct for bipeds and quadrupeds. The cranial end of the isolated spinal cord should be towards the top of the frame. The cords of most quadrupeds should not be oriented horizontally in photographs unless the view is of a lateral surface. Fortunately, protruding lesions (e.g. meningiomas) may be depicted with better modeling in a vertical format. One modeling light, with or without fill-in illumination, is usually suitable. The background and specimen should be rotated a little and the effect on lighting observed through the viewfinder.

Lesions deep in the spinal cord such as hemorrhagic myelomalacia (so-called "hematomyelia") may not be visible at all from the outside, or if visible, not for their entire length. One way to depict these lesions and their location dramatically is to cut uniformly 0.5cm to 1cm wide cross sections of spinal cord, using an extremely sharp razor blade to prevent compression. The cord segments are arranged with their caudal cut surface uppermost in a vertical photographic format, with the most cranial segment to the top of the frame and with the left side of the cord to the left side of the frame. If more than several segments are included, it may be necessary to place them in several rows. Two or three vertical rows can be arranged side by side in a horizontal format. It is better to limit the number of cross sections to two or three, otherwise the viewer's attention is diluted. At the time of photography, accurate records such as a diagram should be made to identify each cord segment.

Longitudinal (midsagittal) sections can be used to emphasize the cranio-caudal direction and the extent of lesions, particularly in the grey matter (e.g. hemorrhagic myelomalacia). Okazaki and Campbell (1979) suggest a cross section at the point of maximum damage to the cord and longitudinal sections through the remainder. If the exact extent of the lesion is not obvious from external examination and the pathologist needs to keep identified cord segments for histopathological examination, 0.5cm wide cross sections can be made at the site of the emergence of the nerve rootlets of each segment and longitudinal sections made through the intervening cord segments. One texture light and a black background is best for color transparencies of cross sections of spinal cord. However, if a close-up photograph of a lesion in a cord segment is to be taken, a dark grey background to de-emphasize the edge of the cord and to allow the eyes to examine the interior of the specimen is more suitable.

Peripheral Nerves

Lesions are rarely visible in peripheral nerves. Exceptions are neurofibromas, damage from trauma such as avulsion of the brachial plexus or neuromas following previous transection. To illustrate their location, neurofibromas, not infrequently seen as multiple neurofibromatosis in cattle, should be photographed *in situ* if possible. Then peripheral nerves should be dissected free and rephotographed. If the lesions are in the cord rootlets, the nerves should be left attached to their spinal cord segments. Similarly, avulsion of the nerves of the brachial plexus is most dramatically presented by photographs of the appropriate cord segments, e.g. C_8-T_2, in dorsal or ventral view to contrast the absence of nerve rootlets on one side with the normal ones on the other. The normal nerves should be cut 1cm to 3cm long, depending on the size of the animal (Mouwen and deGroot, 1982).

Lesions of Marek's disease may be visible grossly in the nerves of birds. In this disease, normal cross striations are replaced by an amorphous grey appearance due to a mononuclear cell infiltrate. These lesions are often only visible in extreme close-ups (RR = 1:1 or RR = 1:2) and often only after the adjacent fascia has been dissected off. Photographs of whole birds showing the nerves can be used for orientation, but these will only rarely show detail. Lesions such as these are difficult to photograph *in situ* because the nerves rarely lie flat to remain within the narrow depth of field available at RR = 1:1. Nerves can be damaged by the injection of medicaments into their vicinity, but only rarely are gross lesions visible. Sometimes, edema, hemorrhage or discoloration of the nerve, adjacent fascia and muscle by a medicament will be sufficiently intense to be visible in a photograph.

Reproductive System

In our necropsy technique, the urinary and female or male reproductive systems are removed *en bloc* after the lateral wall of the pelvis has been removed by sagittal cuts through the pubis to the obturator foramen, from the obturator foramen through the ischium to the arch of the ischium and by a third cut through the "neck" of the ilium, cranial to the acetabulum. The urinary, reproductive, and alimentary (rectum and anus) systems are separated after removal from the pelvis. Displacements such as torsion of the canine uterus should be photographed *in situ* after removal of the lateral pelvic wall (Fig. 4.24).

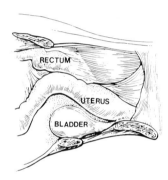

Figure 4.24. View of the pelvic contents after removal of a lateral wall through the pubis and ischium at the obturator foramen and the shaft of the ilium.

Female Reproductive System

After being dissected free of the urinary system and rectum, the female reproductive system is positioned on its ventral surface in a vertical format (Fig. 4.25). In keeping with the anatomic convention of having the cranial portion of the organ system to the top of the frame, the ovaries are at the top and the vulva at the bottom. Placing the long axis of the vagina and uterus horizontally is not satisfactory, because one uterine horn is "above" the other which is a position that does not occur naturally. The female reproductive tract is opened by a dorsal midsagittal incision from the dorsal commissure of the vulva, through the vagina, cervix and uterine body and then along each uterine horn. This reveals the clitoris, cervix, mucosa and nature of the contents of the vagina and uterus. Modeling or texture lighting with or without a fill-in light is required to bring out the detail in exudates or such changes as cystic

glandular hyperplasia. Ovaries can be incised to reveal corpora lutea.
Broad ligaments should be spread to expose thickenings such as thrombosed vessels or exudates from peritonitis. The vertical format is not
only accepted anatomically but is the best lighting position under the
standardized lights.

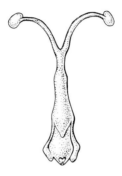

Figure 4.25.

In some cases where it is desired to dramatize the thickness of the
uterine walls such as in a panmetritis, the uterus can be fixed by the
injection of 10% NBF into the lumens of the horn and body and fixation
completed by immersion. Later, cross-sectional slices can be cut to reveal
the thickened walls. Color can be partially restored by immersion in
80%–95% ethanol. Slices should be positioned with the cranial ones to the
top of the frame and in same shape as the uterus (Fig. 4.25), similar to the
arrangement described for cross sections of arteries and veins (Fig. 4.14).

Placenta

Many types of placentitis in animals are characterized by thickening of
the placenta by inflammatory exudates. In ruminants, purulent exudate
may accumulate both in the cotyledons and in the normally transparent
intercotyledonary tissues with the result that the amnion may become
opaque. To demonstrate exudate, texture lighting is required. Changes
in transparency are apparent when the amnion is spread carefully over a
glass with either a black, dark grey or transilluminated background.
Thus, to reveal detail in structures such as amnionic plaques, a combination of texture lighting for surface detail and a background to show
changes in translucency are required. Dark backgrounds are better for
transparencies and light transilluminated ones for monochrome prints.

Mammary Gland

Photographs of *whole* isolated mammary glands of large animals are frequently not very informative, because positioning of such a large non-rigid specimen is difficult. It is better to photograph lesions such as glands with acute mastitis, necrosis, gangrene, tumors and ulceration on the live animal. Canine mammary glands, attached to an ellipse of skin removed by radical mastectomy, are easy to photograph because the glands are smaller and rigid. They should be dissected free of subcutaneous fat to reveal their size and any metastases in lymphatics. Orientation is easy if the surgeon identifies one gland by a suture or leaves the inguinal fat and inguinal lymph node attached. A vertical format with the inguinal fat to the bottom of the frame is anatomically correct, and one modeling light from the top left with reduced fill-in illumination is the preferred lighting.

The conventional method of dissecting mammary glands of both large and small animals is to slice them transversely, in a series, insuring that one incision passes through the teat and cistern to reveal milk or exudate. Acutely inflamed mammary gland, like pneumonic lung, is firm and relatively easy to slice, while normal mammary gland is spongy and difficult to cut. A long straight-bladed knife is required to cut completely through the mammary gland in one slice, for, like other parenchymatous organs, mammary glands are prone to produce specular highlights if the knife cuts leave serrations. The character of the lesion is dramatically presented if the gland has patches of abnormal and normal tissue adjacent to each other. If one gland of a large animal is completely affected, the adjacent normal gland can be included for comparison. Most slices of bovine mammary glands fit into a horizontal format with the teats at the bottom (Fig. 4.26). It is highly desirable to include teats, as these aid in orientating the viewer. Modeling or texture lighting with reduced or no fill-in illumination should be tried.

Teats. Lesions on the external surface of teats or in the sphincter can be photographed during life. Damage to the sphincter with leakage of milk can be dramatically depicted if a stream of milk is pouring from the sphincter. Photographs taken after death have the advantage of better lighting. Teats may be completely removed and photographed with texture lighting to bring out surface detail in lesions such as viral papillomas (warts). If four teats are to be photographed, a vertical format should be used with the cranial pair of teats at the top and the left teats

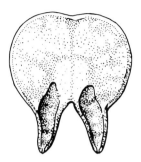

Figure 4.26.

on the left side to avoid confusion in orientation. Lesions in the cistern and teat canal are demonstrated by a longitudinal section of the teat, preferably while it is still attached to the gland.

Male Reproductive System

Photography of lesions on the penis is described under "Urinary System." The penile urethra is opened in the midventral line starting at the urethral orifice. This incision becomes middorsal as the urethra changes direction around the arch of the ischium. The dorsal midsagittal cut is continued through the prostate and into the fundus of the bladder. If the prostate is enlarged sufficiently to obstruct the rectum, this obstruction should be photographed *in situ* after the lateral pelvic wall has been removed. The unincised prostate can be rephotographed in a vertical format with the bladder to the top of the frame (Fig. 4.56). The size and outline of the prostate, as well as changes in texture (for example, those due to cystic glandular hyperplasia or a pyogranulomatous prostatitis from blastomycosis), are revealed better by serial, uniformly wide transverse slices placed one above the other in a vertical format with the most cranial slice at the top of the frame.

Testes and Epididymides. One of the most frequent faults in photography of testes of animals is the failure to orientate the long axes of testes in their correct anatomical positions. These positions are different in different species of domestic animals. Correct orientation is not only desirable but is essential to educate students to recognize these differences. The long axes of testes are vertical in ruminants, horizontal in horses and approximately horizontal with the caudal pole slightly elevated in dogs, cats and pigs (Fig. 4.27). Thus, in a photograph of a single testis, a vertical format should be used for ruminant testes and a horizontal format for individual testes of the dog, cat, or pig. Paired testes of all animals also require a horizontal format (Fig. 4.28), and both testes should be oriented so that either their left or right sides are viewed (Fig. 4.28) and not one left and one right (Fig. 4.29), as this confuses the viewer.

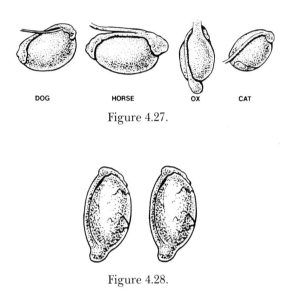

DOG   HORSE   OX   CAT

Figure 4.27.

Figure 4.28.

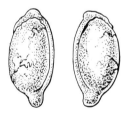

Figure 4.29. This arrangement can be achieved only by viewing a lateral surface of one testis and the medial surface of the other—a confusing mixture.

Many of the problems of slicing and orientating halves of kidney (see "Urinary System") also occur with testes. The halves should be cut completely through with one knife cut so as not to tear the parenchyma when the two pieces are folded back. When a normal testis is cut, the surface bulges and that curvature frequently reflects numerous specular highlights. These are accentuated by serrations from multiple to-and-fro movements of the knife. A single incision with a long sharp-bladed knife is essential, and the prosector must not squeeze the testis, as this will distort the surface. If possible, the longitudinal cut should also transect the epididymis to reveal the cut surfaces of its head, body and tail. Testes from different domestic animals vary considerably in size, and the inclusion of a normal control is helpful for the viewer to appreciate changes in size.

A similar problem also occurs in the orientation of the epididymides of different species (Fig. 4.27). The body of the epididymis is caudal in ruminants and dorsal in most of the other domestic animals. Thus, the epididymis should be on the left or right, or at the top of the frame, respectively. Occasionally, a caudal view of bovine or ovine testis will be required to reveal changes in the shape of an epididymis, particularly of the tail.

Lighting of halved testes usually requires one modeling light, with the surface of the specimen tilted or propped to expose all of it to light. Lighting of whole testes usually requires a main light and a fill-in light to eliminate shadows.

Respiratory System

Upper Respiratory Tract

At necropsy, the larynx, trachea and lungs are removed *en bloc* with the tongue, pharynx, esophagus and heart. The upper respiratory tract may be exposed either by a midsagittal saw cut through the skull to reveal the nasal passages, nasal septum and turbinates or by serial transverse sections 0.5cm–2cm wide, depending on the size of the head. After a midsagittal cut, if the nasal septum is still in place it will have to be removed to allow the underlying turbinates and nasal passage on that side to be examined. This technique is suitable for exposing exudative rhinitis, parasites such as *Oestrus ovis* and neoplasms such as chondrosarcomas, fibrosarcomas or adenocarcinomas arising in the caudal nares and infiltrating into the ethmoid bone and cranial vault. To make serial transverse sections, the whole head should be completely skinned and then sawn on a band saw. Transverse sections reveal the nasal passage, turbinates, and nasal sinuses. Slices are oriented in the same fashion as brain slices (Fig. 4.21), left side on the viewer's left and the most rostral slice at the top of the frame. The technique emphasizes the lack of symmetry due to lesions such as neoplasms of the nasal cavity or sinuses and changes in turbinates, e.g. atrophic rhinitis.

Sawing transverse sections of the head of a large animal can be difficult because teeth have to be cut. Frequently, grease from teeth or saw will be smeared onto the cut surface of the lesion. The surface can be cleaned, but fragile lesions such as adenocarcinomas of the nasal turbinates may be damaged by scrubbing. In such cases, better results can be obtained by first fixing the tissue in 10% NBF for several days, then cleaning the cut surface with towels and a soft brush and finally restoring color with 80%–95% ethanol. Color restoration is adequate for color photography but is particularly useful for black-and-white photography, as the color increases the tonal (grey scale) variations in the lesion thus making a more realistic and interesting monochrome photograph. Fluid exudates from sinusitis will be lost by this technique, and these are best retained and demonstrated by ronguering away the lateral and dorsal walls of the nasal sinuses in the intact skull. Longitudinal and cross-sectional slices should be illuminated by one modeling light alone or with reduced fill-in light.

Larynx and Trachea

The standard necropsy procedure is to open the larynx (Fig. 4.30) and trachea in the dorsal midline from the pharynx to the major bronchi. The walls are spread apart to display the lumen and contents such as edema fluid or inflammatory exudates. The major difficulty is to expose the lumen for photography, as the springy cartilaginous rings tend to return to their normal position. A wide variety of unsuitable props including wooden applicator sticks, pieces of wooden tongue depressors, 1×3 inch glass microscope slides and hypodermic needles have all been used as spreaders, both for the larynx and trachea. The tracheas of small animals and birds have been pinned down and, in some cases, the heads of pins have been larger than the diameter of the trachea. All of these props are distracting and their use should be avoided.

A Gelpi retractor is the least objectionable spreader, although its gleaming stainless steel, even if it has a satin finish, is distracting. If lesions are bilaterally symmetrical, the larynx can be bisected midsagittally to expose the lateral luminal surface (Fig. 4.31). One half can be photographed. The longitudinal axis of a larynx in a standing domestic animal is oblique, between vertical and horizontal. In photographs of a

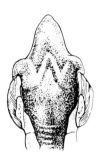

Figure 4.30. Correct anatomical position for viewing the ventral mucosal surface of the larynx. This position requires the use of a vertical camera format.

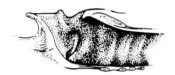

Figure 4.31. Correct position of the larynx when viewing the internal surface after a sagittal cut.

lateral wall, the longitudinal axis of the larynx or trachea should be horizontal (Fig. 4.31).

Exposing the tracheal mucosa is difficult and retractors or props rarely work well. A more suitable method is to excise the dorsal one-third to one-half of the trachea to expose the ventral luminal mucosa and thus eliminate the need for retractors. In a dorsal view, the trachea should be positioned with its long axis vertical. This is the correct anatomic position, but it may be difficult to illuminate the lumen, even with two lamps. Also, lamps in this position will not bring out the texture of exudate. The other alternative is to position the trachea longitudinally and use only one lamp—the left modeling light. The ruler should be placed at the edge of the right side of the horizontal frame, making this the bottom of the photographic frame. Thus, because the light should come from the top and not from below, and because the ruler should be at the bottom of the frame, the transparency can be projected in a vertical format and will appear correctly illuminated.

Changes in shape of the lumen of the trachea, for example, those from congenital abnormalities of the dorsal ligament, are most dramatically depicted in full cross sections. Slices should be cut between cartilaginous rings with an extremely sharp razor blade. Because the normal shape of cross sections of the trachea varies in different species (Fig. 4.32), a normal control of the same species, age and level of the trachea should be included. Rings should be arranged with the most rostral at the top of the frame and the left side of the rings towards the left side of the frame.

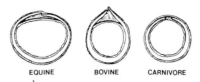

EQUINE   BOVINE   CARNIVORE

Figure 4.32. Transverse section of tracheal rings to illustrate the normal differences in shape between equine, bovine and carnivore rings.

Lack of symmetry of vocal cords as occurs in paralysis of the recurrent laryngeal nerve in equine "roarers" may be demonstrated by standing the isolated larynx vertically on a transilluminated background. The major difficulty is to position the larynx so that the camera views the borders of the vocal cords against a clear background. An alternate technique is to make serial transverse slices across the larynx (Ludwig, 1979a). Both modeling and fill-in lights are required to illuminate cross sections of larynx, although only reduced fill-in may be desirable. The intensity and the effect of the fill-in illumination should be checked in the viewfinder. In the case of asymmetric vocal cords, the top illumination should be half (for color transparencies) to one third (for black and white prints) of the transillumination, so that the outline of the vocal cords stands out in relief against a light grey background.

Lungs

Some lesions are better displayed if the lungs are not allowed to collapse, an event which occurs naturally when the thorax is opened or if there has been a long delay between death and necropsy. To prevent collapse, the glottis may be blocked by a piece of wooden dowel which is tied in place by string. Dowels of different diameter are kept in our necropsy laboratory to fit the glottises of different-sized animals. The trachea of a small laboratory animal may be clamped with hemostats or a bowel clamp. If the lungs have already collapsed, they may be redistended by the intratracheal injection of Jores' solution, sufficient solution being used just to remove the crinkling from the visceral pleura. In small laboratory animals the solution can be injected intratracheally with a syringe and needle. In larger animals, the lungs are suspended vertically and filled with Jores' solution or a fixative such as 10% NBF through the trachea. However, to maintain correct hydrostatic pressure, a variety of procedures have been described and reviewed by Ludwig (1979a). The simplest one is to have the bottle of Jores' solution with its fluid surface 25cm to 30cm above the lungs, which should float in a bath of Jores'. The tube from the bottle is sutured or clamped into the bronchus or trachea. Without redistension, some lesions are not easily seen by the naked eye and are almost invisible in a photograph. Thus 0.5mm–1mm anthracotic foci are strikingly evident in redistended lungs of freshly exsanguinated animals. Also, the contour between pneumonic and normal lung is far better demonstrated if lungs are distended by air or Jores' solution. Redistention takes time but produces optimal specimens for photography. If the lungs are intended for photography only, then Jores' solution should be used. However, if histopathlogical examination is required, lungs should be distended with 10% NBF. These lungs appear similar to those distended with Jores' solution for the first half hour before the 10% NBF changes tissue colors. Initially, reds and pinks become deeper but fade later. The easier and least time-consuming method is to keep the lungs inflated with air by occluding the glottis. This has the advantage of not interfering with the later collection of samples for microbiological or virological examinations. Ludwig (1979a) recommends perfusing one lung and dissecting and culturing the other in the fresh state.

When both lungs are to be photographed from a dorsal view, they should be placed in a vertical format (Fig. 4.33). This position is anatomically correct and is frequently used to depict a pair of lungs in veterinary anatomy textbooks. If lesions are bilaterally symmetrical, the better solution is to photograph the lateral aspect of one lung in a horizontal format (Fig. 4.34). Although unfixed lung is not rigid, it retains relatively normal shape when separated from the thoracic viscera and placed on its medial surface.

The difficulty in photographing lungs of large domestic animals is one of sheer size. The camera may have to be raised to the top of the column to include them in the frame of the camera, and a stepladder may be necessary to allow the operator to focus. An alternative method is to use a wide angle lens, but this should be a last resort because of the distortion it causes. Another alternative is to increase the working distance by removing the specimen background box and placing the lungs on a background on the floor. This will reduce the intensity of illumination on the lungs because they are now 30 inches lower than the usual

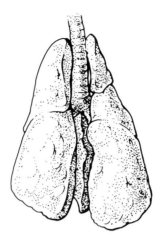

Figure 4.33. Dorsal surface of a lung in its correct anatomic position.

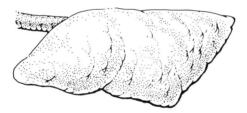

Figure 4.34. Lateral surface of the lung of a quadruped in its correct anatomic position.

position on top of the box and an increase in exposure over the standard-ized exposures will be required.

Problems with the photography of equine and bovine lungs on the floor include:

1. The specimens may not be evenly illuminated with the lights in the standard position. They may have to be repositioned.
2. Legs of the lamp stands may intrude into the field of view of the camera.
3. The results may not justify the trouble. The degree of reduction in size onto the 2 × 2 transparency slide may be so great that little detail will be visible apart from such marked distortion as that due to acute emphysema.

To illuminate a pair of lungs in a vertical format or a single lung in a horizontal format, both modeling and fill-in lamps are required.

Cross sections of lung can show considerable detail, particularly if in pneumonic lungs, normal areas are intermixed with areas of consolidation and emphysema. However, it is extremely difficult to cut a uniformly thick slice of normal or emphysematous lung even with a long straight-bladed knife. Pneumonic lungs are firmer and are easier to slice. Slices should be photographed in an anatomically correct position with caudal surfaces presented to the camera and dorsal surfaces towards the top of the frame (Fig. 4.35). Distribution of lesions in the lung, e.g. extent of a pneumonia (Gogolewski et al., 1987), can be demonstrated by arranging the slices in series with the most cranial at the top of the frame. Lungs which have been fixed by intratracheal perfusion produce excellent cross-sectional slices and show emphysema beautifully, particularly when illuminated with texture lighting. Sufficient time, usually 2–3 days, should be allowed for perfused lungs to harden before transverse slices are made with a long straight-bladed knife such as a disposable brain knife (Fig. 4.20) (see "Equipment"). The cut surface should be illuminated by a modeling or texture light with reduced or no fill-in illumination. Heard and Brackenbury (1962) recommend enhancing the visibility of air spaces by soaking fixed distended lung slices in a 7.5% aqueous solution of barium nitrate for one minute. The slice is then lightly squeezed and transferred to a 10% aqueous solution of sodium sulfate for one minute. Slices of lung are photographed underwater. For this, flat lighting with both lamps at 45° and equidistant from the subject is required.

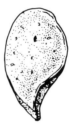

Figure 4.35. Cross section of left lung. The dorsal surface is to the top of the frame and the lateral to the left. This means that a caudal surface is presented.

Skeletal System

Bone

Photographs of the external surfaces of bones are taken to show such obvious changes as exostoses, fractures, neoplasms and discolorations by bilirubin, tetracycline or congenital porphyria. Internal changes to be photographed include reduction in the amount of bone (osteopenia), increased amounts of bone due to diseases such as hereditary osteopetrosis or fluoride toxicosis or changes in the bone marrow due to such changes as neoplasia or hyperplasia. Successful photographs of bones depend on preparation of the specimen. Careful planning is essential, as bone lesions have to be located and their nature evaluated before a decision can be made as to the best method of dissection and presentation. A good example is the demonstration of lesions in joints. Eroded articular surfaces can be revealed simply by opening the joint capsule after cutting through the collateral ligaments and the capsule itself. However, neoplasms of the joint capsule such as a synovioma may be better demonstrated by a sagittal section through the bones forming the joint and the joint capsule. Radiographs and clinical reports should be studied carefully to determine the location, orientation and extent of the lesion and then the results used to plan the best method of dissection.

Preparation of Internal Lesions in Bones. To demonstrate internal lesions, saw cuts through long bones are usually made longitudinally or cross sectionally to show changes in the thickness of the cortex or medullary bone. Changes in the color and amount of bone marrow, in the thickness of epiphyseal cartilages (e.g. rickets) and in metaphyses (e.g. in infarction in neonatal septicemias) are also revealed by longitudinal cuts. Occasionally, long bones must be sawn down their length in a plane other than a sagittal one in order to section a specific lesion, such as a metastatic tumor or through a particular site on the articular cartilage. However, to allow the viewer to orient himself easily, sagittal cuts should be made whenever possible. Sawing longitudinal sections of long bones takes skill. The bone should be completely freed of muscles and tendons which should be cut close to their points of insertion. Care must be taken to ensure that the bone is sawn, on a band saw, in one smooth continuous motion, otherwise saw marks will be made. These are objectionable and will be accentuated further by texture lighting. Bone saws frequently accumulate a dark grease, either from a lubricant or from tissue debris. The grease can be transferred from the blade onto the cut surface of the bone, spoiling the preparation. A similar problem occurs when sawing through hooves and distal phalanges (see "Hooves"). Most of the grease can be removed by scrubbing the bone with a nail brush soaked in physiological saline or .Jores' solution, but the procedure may damage delicate structures such as bone marrow. A better method is to clean the saw blade immediately before use by sawing through 1–2 feet of pine wood such as packing case lumber. Sometimes to demonstrate lesions, it may be desirable to saw a whole leg including skin, soft tissues and bone. Ludwig (1979c) describes a method for human limbs. After fixation, preferably by perfusion with 10% NBF, the leg is frozen and cut on a band saw. Bone dust and frozen fat are removed by brushing, and color is restored by placing the specimen in 80%–95% ethanol.

Preparation of vertebral lesions for photography presents some difficulty, because these lesions frequently involve the spinal cord which must be removed intact for both gross and microscopic examination. A midsagittal section down the isolated vertebral column will reveal changes in vertebral bodies but will destroy the spinal cord. A desirable method would allow both removal of the intact cord and midsagittal sectioning of vertebrae. Removal of the cord via a sagittal cut just lateral to the cord (see "Nervous System") has the disadvantage of destroying articular surfaces (facets) on that side. An alternative method is to expose the cord by sawing the vertebrae horizontally (in quadrupeds) just ventral to the spinal cord. This ventral approach works well, particularly in large animals, as the band saw can be guided down the ventral longitudinal ligament. After removal of the cord, the vertebral bodies, laminae and spinous processes can be sawn midsagittally. This technique preserves intervertebral articular surfaces. A similar approach for primates has been described by Ludwig (1979c). The extent of prolapsed intervertebral disks can be shown by either saggittal or transverse sections through the disks. For comparison, several stages and types of disk protrusion can be included in one photograph (Mouwen and deGroot, 1982).

Internal detail can be seen in bone sections 0.4mm–10mm thick, made transparent by the Spaltenholz clearing method. Photography of this type of specimen on color reversal film, e.g. Ektachrome EPY, tungsten 50 ISO has been described by Hampton and Clarke (1983). They used a slide duplicator with a $3200°K$ light source as a transilluminated background. A 55mm or 35mm lens was used on a bellows on a 35mm camera at RR's of 1.5:1 to 6:1. A lens aperture of f-8 (engraved or relative aperture) gave maximum image quality. This corresponded to effective apertures of f-19 at RR = 1.5:1 and f-56 at RR = 6:1.

Preparation of External Surfaces of Bones. Visualization of lesions of the exterior surfaces of bone requires considerable dissection and preparation. Changes in shape of the bone itself are best revealed after maceration, but changes in color (e.g. those due to periosteal icterus or congenital porphyria) require fresh specimens. For photography of the exterior of fresh bones to be successful, the surface of the periosteum must be cleaned with care. Delicate changes in color such as those due to bilirubin will be lost within hours of exposure. Also, the periosteum itself will dry quickly and lose its glistening "bloom." Thus, for photography, long bones should be cleaned of attached muscles and tendons quickly and delicately, *not* washed in water or Jores' solution and photographed immediately. If this delay between death and necropsy has been sufficient to allow hemoglobin imbibition to occur, bones will be discolored red and photographs will be dull and uninteresting. Osteomalacia and rickets can result in soft bones which can be easily distorted by bending or twisting. This defect can be demonstrated in photographs by distorting the bone held in gloved hands and photographing against a black background to accentuate the outline.

Maceration of Bones. Maceration techniques have been briefly reviewed by Armed Forces Institute of Pathology (1957) and Ludwig (1979c). The methods basically depend upon bacterial, thermal, or chemical removal of tissues. Bacterial decomposition is best done in deep covered pots filled with warm water. The method is cheap, easy, malodorous and slow (Wagner and Nuckolos, 1936). Some techniques recommend fluid from a previous vat to provide the bacterial inoculum. Thermal methods include use of warm water at about 33°C with sodium hydroxide added daily to make the water distinctly alkaline (Rhea, 1922), simmering over a low fire or autoclaving well ossified and very strong bones. One chemical method uses "antiforman" which incorporates a 6% solution of hypochlorite (Rosenthal, 1948). After simmering in hot water (56°C) for 4 to 6 hours, depending on its size, the specimen is immersed and agitated in warm (45°C) 6% hypochlorite solution for 3 to 5 hours.

Photography of Bones. Bones should be photographed in their correct anatomic position which means that long bones should be vertical (Fig. 4.36). Many vertically mounted cameras can be used only with the camera in a horizontal format. The result is that incorrect orientation of long bones and their joints in a horizontal format is a very common defect in photographs. Another photographic problem is that long bones are not of uniform thickness. Thus, they need to be propped up, to raise the surface (either cut or external) to be photographed parallel to the film plane. A vertically mounted camera is not the optimal method of photographing the exterior of many bones. It does not lend itself to flexible positioning of the specimen, to flexible lighting or to selecting the best angle of view, particularly of bones with irregular outlines such as the skull and vertebrae. A studio with a camera on a tripod or stand, versatile lighting and separate background lighting is required for optimal results. The specimen should be supported on a stand that can be rotated, tilted, or both, to obtain the optimal view.

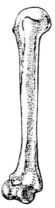

Figure 4.36.

An oblique view of the dorsal and lateral surfaces of the skull or several vertebrae (Fig. 4.37) or the sacrum allows the viewer to see both dorsal and lateral surfaces which is far more informative than a strictly lateral or dorsal view. Lesions on an articular surface of a long bone such as the proximal end of a humerus may be more comprehensible when viewed from a point dorsal and cranio-lateral to that surface. In other words, the specimen would be rotated and tilted to give the best view. Hence, photographs of complicated bones are best taken by a biological photographer who has both skill and an adequately equipped studio.

The majority of macerated specimens will be "high key" (the photographic term for a subject where the tonal range is very short with the majority of the tones being very light). Retention of detail in monochrome photographs of high-key subjects takes considerable skill in

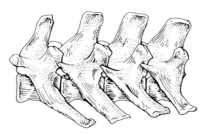

Figure 4.37. Vertebrae. An oblique view (in this case, along a caudal, ventral and medial axis) is far more informative than a dorsal or lateral view. The relationship between vertebrae is revealed better.

lighting and processing of the negative and print. For transparency photographs, skulls and vertebrae can be placed directly on a black velvet background. Long bones can be supported vertically on a black vertical spike inserted into, or glued to, the lower articular surface. In black-and-white photographs, the props can be obliterated from the negative by photographic opaque to produce a white background.

Photographs of Bones for Measurement. If bones (for example, long bones of experimental animals) are to be photographed for comparison or measurement, it is essential to take precautions which include:

1. preservation of all anatomic landmarks so that an accurate and measurable outline is retained.
2. inclusion of a control bone for comparison.
3. control of perspective by using a long focal length lens (105mm, 135mm, 150mm for a 35mm camera). Because of the smaller angles of acceptance, their working distances are longer and this prevents distortion. Williams (1984) suggests using a "very long focal length lens."
4. careful leveling of the plane of the bone so that it is parallel to the film plane, again to prevent distortion due to "keystoning."
5. inclusion of a scale close to the bone and also in the same plane as that of the bone, so that both these subjects are in focus in the plane of principal focus of the lens.
6. A black box background (Martinsen, 1968) to emphasize the outline of the bone.

Joints

Joints can be extremely difficult to photograph because:
1. Different types of lesions require different dissection techniques,

depending on whether the lesions involve the articular surfaces (e.g. erosions, exudates) or joint capsules (e.g. villous hyperplasia).

2. Correct anatomic orientation frequently requires the use of props and clamps which are difficult to mask off so that the background is plain.

3. Lighting to convey differences in shape and texture of joint surfaces in monochrome prints requires skill.

Lesions in joints may be on the joint capsule (e.g. villous hyperplasia or arthritis) or on the articular surfaces (e.g. erosions, exudate) or proliferative lesions of the bone itself, or there can be lesions at all three sites.

Techniques Used to Dissect Joints.

These are:

1. A sagittal cut through the bones of joints such as the femoro-tibial (Fig. 4.38), carpal and tarsal joints to expose the joint capsule, articular cartilages, synovial membrane, physes and diaphyses (Ludwig, 1979c). This technique works well if the joints contain exudate or neoplasms (e.g. fibrosarcoma or synovioma of the joint capsule) but is not the most suitable to show changes on articular surfaces. It is critical that the bones be cut cleanly without saw marks and that the saw itself be free of grease as described previously.
2. Disarticulation of the joint. Joints should be opened by cutting the surrounding muscle, tendons and ligaments, but, to avoid any chance of artifacts, the knife should not enter the joint cavity. This insures that changes on the articular cartilages are genuine and not caused by the prosector. Also, this technique prevents contamination of exudates or fluid which can then be cultured. To minimize distractions in a photograph, adjacent muscles and tendons should be completely stripped off bones without damaging the periosteum.
3. Macerate bones to show exostoses.

Thus, the prosector has to determine which type of lesion is present and how it can best be demonstrated before dissection is started. Sometimes, it is necessary to decide which lesions are to be emphasized. An erosive arthritis can be demonstrated by disarticulating the joint, but arthritis with ankylosis obviously cannot be demonstrated in this way. Alternative approaches are to macerate the bones to reveal the ankylosis or make a sagittal cut to expose the site of the ankylosis. Because of limitations of

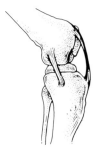

Figure 4.38.

what can be revealed by dissection, photographs of radiographs should be used in conjunction with gross photographs in lectures.

Before opening joints by disarticulation, all muscles, tendon and any debris should be removed from the exterior. If it is necessary to remove contamination from the exterior of the bone, this should be washed away with physiological saline or Jores' solution. Once the joint is opened, any tags of tissue along the joint capsule should be trimmed away neatly and the photograph taken with minimal delay. Normal articular cartilage has a characteristic bluish-grey bloom which is lost quickly if the specimen dries or even if it is blotted. It is essential to avoid artifacts such as knife cuts or knicks in the cartilage, as such artifacts can be confused with fragmentation or erosions.

Photographic Problems of Bones and Joints. The chief problems in the photography of bones and joints are:

1. Maintaining correct anatomic orientation.
2. Obtaining an unobtrusive background free of the clutter of props and clamps used to hold the bone in correct orientation.
3. Lighting to bring out texture and modeling.

1. **Anatomic Orientation.** Because many vertically mounted cameras can be used only with the camera in a horizontal format, orientation of long bones and their joints has often been incorrect in photographs. Another problem is that if long bones are not of uniform thickness, they need to be propped up to raise either the cut or external surface parallel to the film plane. Even more difficult to orient are the articular surfaces of long bones. These generally have to be held by some type of clamp. Convention is to have the cranial (anterior) border to the top of the frame with the left side of the joint correctly oriented to the left side of the frame (Fig. 4.39). Because most joints are quite small, photographs

have to be taken with RR's between 1:1 and 1:3 and thus depth of field is shallow. Joint surfaces are often uneven due to facets and condyles. To keep these in focus when depth of field is shallow, the specimen may have to be oriented so that the plane of focus is through the middle of the depth of the articular surface. This may require slight tilting of the articular surface away from the anatomical position. A versatile clamp such as a laboratory stand is required to hold long bones so that their articular surfaces can be photographed. Stands have the disadvantage that they require space on the photographic background and may cast shadows. Also, the clamp itself may be visible in the photograph.

Figure 4.39. Articular surface of tibia. The cranial surface is to the top of the frame.

2. **Background.** For black-and-white negatives, the simplest procedure is to photograph the specimen with a large-format negative and opaque the clamps and background out of the negative to obtain a white background in the print. If a black background is required to emphasize the shape of the outline of the bone or joint, the image of the clamp can be scraped off the negative.

Control of background clutter is even more difficult in transparencies. Unfortunately, there are few good solutions. These include:

1. Orient the shaft of the long bone so that it slopes out of the field of view. This will mean that the clamp can also be out of the field of view but will result in the camera having a slightly oblique view of the articular surface and some of the shaft. The presence of the shaft can be minimized by framing closely around the articular surface. This technique will be satisfactory where extensive lesions are present over the articular surface and the field of view is chosen to control the amount of background. In other words, the field is selected to minimize background rather than to choose the optimal position for viewing lesions.
2. Paint clamps dull black and use a black background. Clamp will still be visible but less obtrusive.
3. Drape the clamp with a disposable black velvet or rubber background. One method is to pierce a hole in the drape and insert the

shaft of the bone through so that the drape covers all of the field except the end of the bone. Rogers (1976) and Daguid and Ollerenshaw (1962) placed elastic around holes in white cotton sheets and black flannel respectively as drapes for photography of the plantar surfaces of feet of human patients. Similar drapes could be made for use with bones. Any folds in drapes, except black velvet, will be visible and distracting. Macerated bones which are clean can be draped with black velvet. For fresh specimens, disposable black velvet remnants can be used. Fine bone dust from the macerated bones will have to be removed from the velvet (e.g. by a blast of compressed air). Draping with black velvet has the advantage of masking off the shaft which would be visible but out of focus in the field of view.

4. Hold the shaft in a gloved hand. This procedure has been described for the heart. Orientation of the articular surface can be optimal, and clean well-fitting natural latex gloves are relatively unobtrusive. As there will be movement of the specimen, exposures must be extremely short and preferably made by electronic flash.

5. Cut the shaft of the bone transversely close to the neck at such an angle that the bone will stand on its cut end. The balance may be precarious and the direction of cut which allows the bone to balance may not be one which results in the plane of the articular surface being parallel to the film plane (i.e., in the plane of focus). Small pieces of modeling clay can be used to "stick" the bone to the background.

6. Carpal bone. If the carpus is affected, as for example in a generalized degenerative joint disease, a row of carpal bone is easy to orient and photograph. Because the bones are of relatively uniform thickness, the surface of these bones is almost flat and they are easily positioned under the camera. The background can be tilted and rotated to obtain the best lighting angle, usually with one lamp to give texture lighting. Articular surfaces are usually a very light grey and exposure has to be accurate, as latitude in transparencies with such a light subject is usually less than ½ stop.

3. **Lighting of Bones and Joints.** The standardized lamps work quite well for photography of many lesions on articular surfaces and on the cut and external surfaces of bones. When modeling or texture lighting is required to illuminate flat surfaces, the 60° modeling light or the 80° texture light should be used. However, some type of fill-in illumination

is usually required with whole bones, but the full output of the fill-in light of the standardized lights may be excessive and should be reduced by one of the methods described under "Lighting." Blaker (1977e) recommends that long bones be illuminated by the same technique used for cylindrical objects which is to light them from one end by direct or diffuse light. He feels that cross lighting makes shadows difficult to control and the edge nearest the light merges with a light or white background, and cross lighting causes bands of light and dark along the length of the axis of the cylinder. This may be true of metallic cylinders, but we have not had this problem with fresh bones on a dark grey or black background. Lighting from one end can be done under the standardized lamps but with a couple of departures from the normally recommended procedure. A long bone would have to be positioned horizontally, an anatomically incorrect position, with the upper extremity of the bone towards the main (modeling) light. This would cause little difficulty if no fill-in illumination was used. The ruler would have to be placed along the edge of the right-hand side of the frame (i.e. the anatomic bottom of the frame). If no fill-in illumination was used, there would be no illumination from under the specimen ("spook" lighting) and the ruler would not cast a shadow. However, if deep shadows are present on the lower extremity or under some lesion, fill-in illumination will have to be added. To prevent the appearance of spook lighting, a minimal amount of fill-in illumination should be used and care should be taken by positioning the fill-in lamp or by using a suitable background to ensure that the ruler does not cast a shadow into the picture. The best approach is to place the specimen in its correct anatomic position which is vertical for long bones, illuminate it with the standardized lights and then rotate the specimen and background through about 30° clockwise and counterclockwise to see if the visibility of the lesions is improved. It is likely that positioning a long bone so that the main light is directed down its axis is only rarely required.

Unmacerated dissected bones can be stored in Jores' solution and forwarded to a biological photographer. This works well with most specimens, but fibrinous or purulent exudates will be washed away and articular cartilages changed from grey to pink. Clean macerated specimens which require expert photographic skill to light successfully should be sent to a biological photographer with a well-equipped studio.

Skin and Hooves

For convenience, photography of both necropsy and clinical specimens will be described here. Requirements for photography of skin have been summarized by the statement of Hansell and Ollerenshaw (1962) that it is of the utmost importance to show: (1) the general distribution and extent of lesions and (2) details of lesions themselves. In human dermatology it is usually necessary to take full- and half-length figures to show distribution of lesions and also 1:1 (life-sized) views of representative areas which need not include orienting landmarks to reveal detail. Hansell (1947) states that photographs of skin lesions are often inadequate because of a distressing compromise between the close-up and general views. He commends the example of motion pictures where a general view is followed by a close-up to reveal detail. When there is only one lesion, sometimes it is possible to include sufficient surrounding area with orienting anatomic landmarks to allow the viewer to estimate size (Hansell, 1947). These remarks are even more applicable to large animal dermatology where photographs of the whole animal will reveal little or no detail.

Preparation of Skin. Human patients are frequently smeared with ointments which may obscure the lesion, and thus cleaning of the area is essential (Hansell, 1947). Light oils and ether can be used for cleaning. Similarly, animal subjects should be cleaned, but cleaning must be gentle so as not to dislodge scales and crusts (Hansell, 1947) and so alter the character of the lesion. Hansell (1947) also recommends applying a trace of light oil to the skin of human subjects and uses a 5%–10% paraffin oil in ether to impart a luster to the surface. For animal patients, oil should be tried only after photographs have been taken without it. The biggest problem in veterinary pathology is to see the lesion because of its being obscured by hair coat. If there is depilation, photographs should be taken to record this and then the hair removed by clippers to reveal the nature of the skin lesions themselves.

Lighting. Evaluation of transparencies of skin lesions in clinical cases shown at conferences reveals that in many of these lighting is poor. The major faults are light coming from below—"spook" lighting, flat lighting without texture of modeling and deep, heavy shadows. Hansell and Ollerenshaw (1962) emphasize that in skin photography, rendition of "texture is of prime importance" and this is particularly true of veterinary dermatology, as, unlike human caucasian skin, many of the color differences seen in skin lesions are obscured by hair coat and pigmentation in animals. Some of the findings of Salthouse (1958) on the reflection of light from lightly and heavily pigmented human skins are of direct application to veterinary dermatology. In lightly pigmented skins, light penetrates through the epidermis and dermis and is reflected by the surface of the stratum corneum, by the various layers of the epidermis, the dermis and even by the subcutis. However, in heavily pigmented skins, light is reflected only from the surface of the stratum corneum, since most rays which penetrate the epidermis are absorbed by the pigment. In photographic terms, this means that the light forming the image from light-colored skins is a mixture of light reflected from the surface and light reflected from the different layers of the skin (epidermis, dermis, subcutis), and thus both differences in color and texture can be seen. The situation is very different with black or very dark skins. The only light forming the image is that reflected from the surface, and thus to produce any detail, it is necessary to use texture lighting (Fig. 3.5). Also, because little or no light is reflected from the deeper layers of the skin, those rays are not available to act as fill-in illumination for the shadows cast by the texture light. This results in an increase in contrast with very deep shadows. Thus, for the successful photography of dark skin, texture and balanced fill-in lighting must be used (Fig. 4.7). This presents a considerable photographic challenge. The problem of recording texture in photographs of light-colored human skin was overcome by a completely different approach by Callender (1974). Instead of using texture lighting to reveal surface detail, he reduced the translucency of the skin and emphasized texture by coating the skin with either a hand cream containing carbon or petroleum jelly containing black poster powder. One of these was smeared on the skin and then rubbed off with absorbent cotton until the black pigment remained only in the depressions between the ridges. An even diffuse light was used, and photographs clearly revealed the outline and patterns of the ridges and valleys. The problem of texture lighting is further compounded by the difficulty in calculating correct exposure. Reflecting light meters or cameras metering TTL or OTF are calibrated on the assumption that the subject is "average" and reflects 18 percent of the light falling on it. Thus, these meters will not give correct exposure with very light and very dark subjects. The former will be darkened and the latter lightened in the photograph.

It is useful to review the requirements for successful photography in clinical veterinary dermatology. These are:

1. The use of a texture light and fill-in lights to record detail and yet at the same time provide uniform illumination. This can be difficult to achieve in large animals.
2. Short exposure to "freeze" movement, usually implying the use of electronic flash.
3. Unobtrusive backgrounds which are particularly difficult to obtain with dark-skinned or dark-haired animals. Preferably, the background should have its own illumination to eliminate shadows cast by the subject.
4. Selection of a field of view containing a single lesion and yet to allow viewer orientation and include detail of color, texture, depth and size of the lesion (Smialowski and Currie, 1960b).

Because of the natural lack of cooperation by animals, the photographer is left with little alternative but to use lightweight electronic flash units. Over the years, several alternatives have been described to try to obtain some texture or modeling with electronic flash units. Methods have basically fallen into two classes: a single flash mounted to the side of the camera to produce some modeling but with a relatively small lighting angle (15°–30°) so that no fill-in illumination was required. This is the basis of the technique described by McGavin (1961) for photography of eyes and Kutscher (1978) for photography of skin. He mounted a small electronic flash head on a variably positionable 18 inch swivel rod to the left of his 2-1/4 × 2-1/4 reflex camera. This enabled him to change the lighting angle to reveal texture in caucasian skin and also to obtain even illumination and predictable results. The swivelling flash arm, which was custom made, screwed into the tripod mount on the base of the camera and could be moved to adjust the lighting angle. The flash head was mounted on the rod, and the power pack was held over the photographer's shoulder. Modern flash units of similar light output are lightweight, compact and fit directly onto the rod and do not require a separate power pack.

Kutscher and Dehner (1983) modified the technique to suit a 35mm single-lens-reflex camera. A ring-flash (Olympus Model T-10) was mounted directly on the 55mm macro-lens of an Olympus OM-2N camera with a power pack positioned in the top shoe. The camera and an Olympus T-32 flash head were mounted on a modified Cullmann macro-extension rod (Cullmann GMBH, Langenzenn, F.D.R.) designed to allow the distance between flash head and camera to be changed by sliding the rod with the flash mounted on its end. The distance to which this rod should be extended for each RR was marked on the rod. The flash reflector was mounted on an adjustable mount at 45° to the optical axis of the camera. Thus, modeling light supplied by the laterally mounted flash was augmented by even fill-in illumination from the ring flash on the camera's lens. Exposure was monitored automatically by two silicone blue cell sensors in the camera's mirror box. These faced the film plane and read the light reflected from the film and automatically adjusted the length of the discharge of the flash units to ensure correct exposure. This technique allows standardized lighting and exposure with fields of view from RR = 1 to RR = 1:6 (field sizes of $1 \times 1\text{-}1/2$ to 6×9 inches for a 35mm camera). As described under "Lighting," automatic exposure flash units can be badly misled by very light or very dark subjects, as the flash unit is calibrated on the assumption that the "average" subject reflects 18 percent of incident light. Other manufacturers now market "outfits" designed to give modeling and fill-in illumination in close-up photography. The ability of the TTL–OTF metering to automatically control the duration of both the modeling and fill-in flash units has been the basis of its success.

For veterinary clinical dermatology there are two useful approaches, both based on the use of twin matched dedicated flash units. In the first method, one flash unit, usually the left, acts as a main or modeling light and is hand-held at a 30°–50° lighting angle. The other flash unit mounted on the camera is operated at reduced ($1/4$ to $1/8$) output as a fill-in light. This has been described in detail under "Equipment." The procedure works well for large fields such as photographs of small domestic animals down to RR = 1:6 (field size of 6×9 inches with a 35mm camera). At larger RR's it becomes more convenient to mount the flash units directly onto a Lepp rod (see "Equipment"). With this equipment (Fig. 4.40) the modeling light is mounted at 45° on an extension rod and the fill-in light at $1/4$ output is mounted close to the lens rim. Exposure can be controlled either by TTL–OTF metering or the unit can be calibrated by trial. Once calibrated, the basic exposure has to be altered only if the reflectivity of the subject is not average. This usually amounts to closing the aperture $1/2$ stop for very light subjects, opening $1/2$ to 1 stop for dark hair coats, and $1\text{-}1/2$ stops for very dark to black coats.

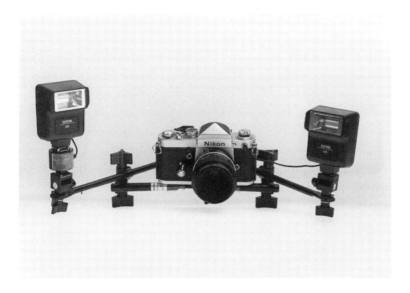

Figure 4.40. Camera with two matched flash units mounted on a Lepp rod. One unit is the main light (modeling or texture) and the other with its output reduced is the fill-in lamp. Courtesy of Doctor L. J. LeBeau and *Journal of Biological Photography.*

When the Lepp rod is not used, placing the main light at 30°–50° above and 30°–50° to the side (usually the left) can be done by the photographer for subjects at distances of up to 3 feet. However, at longer working distances, the photographer's arm is too short and hence an assistant is needed to hold this light. The power output of the fill-in flash may have to be reduced to ⅛ from the usual ¼ output, if the modeling light is sufficiently further from the subject than the fill-in flash. Our results with a Pentax Super Program camera and two Pentax AF 200T dedicated flash units using TTL–OTF metering has been good with Ektachrome 200 film except for very light and black subjects where exposure has been incorrect. For these subjects, the exposure has to be modified by changing the film speed rating on the dial of the camera. This new rating is determined by trial. With our equipment, "average" subjects were correctly exposed with Ektachrome 200 film with the camera ISO dial set at 200, but ISO ratings of 125 and 320 gave correct exposure for white and black skins, respectively. The only other alternative to changing the film's rating is not to use the TTL–OTF exposure control but to use the flash units in a manual mode. In other words, the full output of the flash units is used and exposure is determined by trial for subjects of different reflectivity by taking a series of photographs at different apertures. This method is more reliable for subjects which are not "average."

For monochrome photography, Salthouse (1958) found that rashes on heavily pigmented human skin were revealed better on panchromatic emulsions by the use of a red filter. For lightly pigmented skins, a blue filter gave better results. The twin-flash technique works well in black-and-white photography. The selection of a film is partially controlled by the working lens aperture for a specific film and distance. This is explained in the manufacturer's literature on the use of dedicated flash units. We have had good results with Plus X Pan film (Fig. 4.41) developed in Kodak D-76 developer diluted 1 + 1 as described below in "Cadaver Photography."

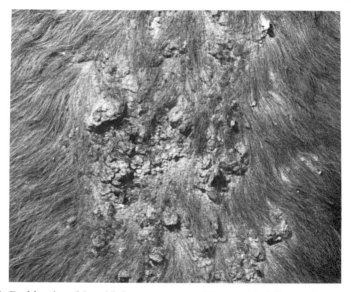

Figure 4.41. Red bovine skin with keratoses caused by atomic fallout, photographed with two matched dedicated flash units. The modeling flash on full output was held above and to the left of the camera. The fill-in flash operating a ¼ output was positioned on the camera. The exposure was controlled by the TTL–OTF metering of the camera.

Backgrounds. Backgrounds for clinical subjects are discussed under "Clinical Photography." As for all backgrounds, these should be plain and unobtrusive. Surgical drapes are frequently used, but they are rarely suitable. The prominent green or blue-green color and texture as well as distracting folds are very obtrusive (Fig. 2.12).

Skin of Cadavers. Unless special precautions are taken, photographs of skin lesions on animal cadavers can be disappointing unless the animals are recently dead. When cadavers are placed in a refrigerator, the hair coat frequently becomes wet or matted. Also, at euthanasia or death, blood or feces may contaminate the hair. If the hair is later washed, the character of the lesions may be altered, e.g. by removal of crusts. Thus, before necropsy, every care should be taken to prevent wetting or soiling of the skin. Another cause of poor results is the extreme difficulty in positioning the body so that the lesions can be lighted suitably by texture lighting. Also, skin lesions may appear unnatural once muscles either lose tone and become flaccid or stiffen in rigor mortis. The wisest procedure is to photograph skin lesions during life, euthanatize the animal without damage to the lesion and rephotograph immediately. Photographs taken postmortem are frequently technically better because of better lighting, but, to the trained observer, there may be a significant departure from the appearance seen during life. Necropsy photographs of lesions such as warts or stephanofilarial dermatitis on isolated pieces of bovine skin can be good. However, such skin pieces should be kept small, because large completely flat areas of skin do not occur on the live animal and thus appear unnatural in photographs. Deep lesions such as epidermoid cysts and furuncles should be sectioned and the cut surface of the skin illuminated by texture lighting.

Hooves

These are frequently extremely dirty and need to be cleaned by hosing and gentle scrubbing with a nail brush and water or physiological saline before dissection. To facilitate photography, the leg of a cadaver can be amputated at the metacarpo-phalangeal (fetlock) joint, carpus or tarsus, depending on the size of the animal. If lesions are on the lateral, medial or cranial surfaces, the leg is relatively easy to position. Lesions on the soles of hooves are much more difficult to position for photography. The equine hoof contains the third phalangeal bone (P_3) and a portion of the second phalangeal bone (P_2). So that the sole can be propped into a position visible to the camera, the hoof may have to be detached by sawing transversely through the shaft of P_2. Alternatively, as described for photography of articular surfaces of long bones (see "Skeletal System"), a laboratory clamp covered by a disposable black velvet drape can be used to hold the leg. Elasticized holes in white sheets (Rogers, 1976) and in black velveteen (Daguid and Ollerenshaw, 1962) as used in the photography of human feet could also be used. Lesions in the interdigital cleft of cloven-footed animals will be visible only after the "claws" have been separated. Remarks applied previously to the use of makeshift retractors apply here, and the least objectionable method is to use hands covered by clean surgical gloves or a Gelpi surgical retractor.

Lesions on the internal wall of the hoof can be revealed either by removal of the hoof by maceration or by sagittal section through the hoof. The technique for sawing bones has already been described (see "Skeletal System"). Hooves attached to the leg should always be orientated vertically which is their normal anatomic position (Fig. 4.42). For comparison purposes, a normal specimen should be included. Ventral rotation of P_3 secondary to laminitis is dramatically depicted if sagittal sections of affected and normal equine phalanges are included side by side in the same photograph. Texture lighting, usually with little if any fill-in lighting, is required.

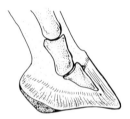

Figure 4.42.

Ears

Ears should always be photographed in a vertical position, using a vertical format for one ear and a horizontal format for two. Photographs of dry gangrene with very dark necrotic areas may need a light grey background. A black background is unsuitable because of inadequate contrast between the specimen and background. Modeling lighting is required. The amount of fill-in illumination necessary will depend on the depth of the shadows and cavities.

Special Senses

Eye

The basic concerns of photography of the external eye of human patients have been described by Stenstrom (1978). These are: accurate depiction of the location of lesions, control of the location, shape and size of specular highlights (catch lights) on the cornea from the light source, and the best camera angle to reveal lesions. Because most patients with eye lesions have photophobia, ambient light levels and focusing lights from flash units should be as dim as possible. This is particularly important in attempting to obtain cooperation from animals. In a room routinely used for ophthalmological examination, the light should be fitted with dimmers. Frequently, too high magnifications RR's = 1 and slightly less are used. These may give excellent detail in the lesion, but its exact location may not be evident from the photograph. Therefore, one photograph should be taken at a suitable RR which allows the inclusion of both lateral and medial canthi to reveal the location of lesions. Hidden lesions, for example, those on the lid conjunctiva, will have to be exposed by everting the lid. This can be done with fingers (preferably gloved and with the minimum amount of the fingers in the photograph) or by cotton-tipped applicators pressed onto the skin a few millimeters from the conjunctival-skin junction to evert the lid. Fletcher (1984) recommends that human patients be photographed at fixed RR's— 1:10, 1:6 for both eyes, a single eye and eyebrow at 1:2 and lesions on a single eye at 1:1. These recommendations can be used for photography of primate eyes, but the eyes of most domestic animals do not look forward and thus photographs of both eyes in the one frame are either not possible or not useful.

Apart from the standardized views, the angle of the camera's optical axis should be selected to reveal the character of the lesion (Stenstrom, 1978). Therefore, the location of lesions on the periorbital skin are revealed best by a "straight-on," i.e. at right angles to a plane through the surface of the eye and the periorbital skin. However, distortions of the cornea (e.g. by keratoconus, exophthalmus) or the nature of protruding lesions on the lids (e.g. keratoses and tumors) will be more clearly revealed in a side view.

One of the major problems in photography of the eye is the presence of the catch-light on the cornea. This can obscure corneal lesions or can be so obtrusive as to detract attention from a lesion. The classic example of the latter is the distracting doughnut-shaped catch-light produced by ringlights. For this reason and because they give a flat even illumination without any modeling, ringlights should not be used for photography of external eyes. The catch-light should be as small as possible, and this can be done easily by the use of a flash unit with a small-diameter reflector. Fortunately, many flash units today have small reflectors and yet sufficient output. Finally, the catch-light should be positioned away from any corneal lesion. This can be done by placing the flash unit on the side of the camera opposite to the one with the lesion. Fletcher (1984) recommends mounting the flash unit on a swivel arm which can be rotated to the left or right of the camera and attaching a small light source (e.g. a penlight) to the flash reflector so that the location of the catch-light on the cornea can be seen.

Lesions in the eye or the periorbital skin are usually best photographed during life (Fig. 4.43). With the advent of ophthalmological cameras, excellent photographs of eyes are quite commonplace. Although photographing the eye of an uncooperative live animal can be frustrating, results can be excellent. On the other hand in photographs of dead animals, eyes usually look "dead" due to a dilated iris or autolysis having produced a cloudy cornea. Also, positioning can be difficult. The optimal procedure is to photograph the eye during life and then later, if possible, at necropsy.

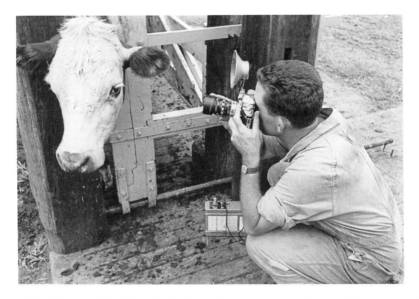

Figure 4.43. Photography of ocular lesions of a range steer using a reflex camera with a 105mm lens, automatic extension tubes and an electronic flash unit mounted to the side. Courtesy of the Editor, *Australian Veterinary Journal.*

Live animal. McGavin (1961) described the standardization of exposures at several RR's for a SLR camera with an electronic flash unit. The basis of the method was to select several RR's, and thus different-sized fields of view and standardized exposure, after angling the flash unit to give even illumination (Fig. 4.44). To take a photograph at a specific RR, angle the flash bracket to a pre-marked position, select the correct aperture and expose after making allowance for any departure from average reflectivity of the specimen. So that the catch-light from the flash can be positioned so that it does not obscure lesions on the cornea, the bracket should be able to be positioned either to the left or the right of the camera. This will require that it be calibrated (Fig. 4.44) for both positions. Since the article was published in 1961, automatic extension tubes (i.e. extension tubes which still allow the diaphragm to close automatically), macro-lenses and automatic exposure for flash units have become available.

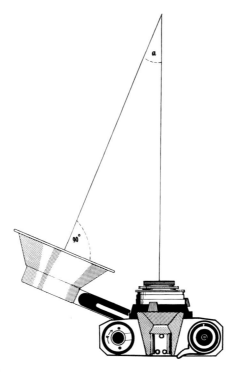

Figure 4.44. The angle of the flash bar (lighting angle) is determined by trial. The flash should point at the center of the subject in focus at a predetermined ratio of reproduction (R:R), e.g. RR = 1:3. Courtesy of the Editor, *Australian Veterinary Journal.*

The twin dedicated flash units with TTL–OTF exposure control can be used for this type of photography, no doubt with better rendition of texture. However, the use of a single flash unit mounted to the side of the camera has some advantages in the photography of eyes. Reflections of the flash, so-called the catch lights in the corneas, are a problem because they may obscure or be confused with lesions. Two flash units produce two catch-lights which are even less desirable. Also, in the photography of unbroken animals such as range cattle, the equipment depicted in Figure 4.43 produced good results with some modeling (Fig. 4.45). Any additional flash units or assistance to hold them would cause these animals to be even less cooperative. The single-flash technique has proved to be highly reliable with thousands of exposures and has produced uniformly good results. A single dedicated flash unit could be used to meter the exposure automatically, but variation in the reflectivity of the periorbital skin may confuse the meter and lead to incorrect exposure. This type of photography is an example where standardization of exposure with a small self-contained flash unit is the best approach.

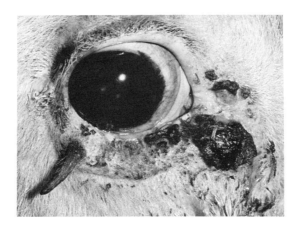

Figure 4.45. Bovine ocular squamous cell carcinoma and keratoses on eyelid photographed as in Figure 4.43. Courtesy of the *Australian Veterinary Journal.*

Difficulties include:

1. Too short a working (lens-subject) distance. The importance of this is the danger of large animals to the operator. Also, the proximity of the operator can annoy the animal. Strangely, some animals blink as they see the finger squeeze the shutter release. The obvious answer is to increase the working distance by using a 105, 135 or 150mm lens on a 35mm camera, but there is a penalty. Because the flash unit is mounted on a bracket attached to the camera, the flash-subject distance is also increased, reducing the amount of light reaching the subject. Thus, a more powerful and probably heavier flash unit may be necessary to allow the use of small

apertures such as *f*-16. The increased working distance also reduces the lighting angle (Fig. 4.44), producing flatter lighting and less modeling. A 105mm lens is a good compromise, but its working distance is too short to guarantee the safety of an operator working with a fractious animal.

2. Lack of cooperation of the animal in opening its eye. This can happen if the patient has photophobia. Unhappily, forcibly opening eyes with fingers causes distorted, misshapen lids as well as introducing the distraction of fingers. Sometimes a patient will cooperate by opening its eye in a dim light or if its head is in a relatively normal position.
3. Lesions obscured by pus, debris and flies.

Necropsy Eye Specimens. The most natural appearance is obtained by excising a wide margin of periorbital skin along with the eyeball. An isolated eyeball appears stark and unnatural. An attempt should be made to arrange the eyeball and palpebral fissure in an approximately normal relationship. Exudate and debris should be washed off the periorbital skin with physiological saline to reveal underlying lesions.

Isolated eyeballs should be photographed in their correct anatomical position. As the corneas will be facing the camera, the left eyeball should be on the right and the right eye on the left and the dorsal surface of the eyes at the top of the frame. A horizontal field is most suitable for photography of two eyeballs. Details of the preparation of internal lesions of eyes for gross specimen photography has been described under "Color Restoration." However, in macrophotography of eye sections, the convention is to position the eye with its optical axis vertical and the cornea towards the top of the frame (Reese, 1956; Yanoff and Fine, 1975).

Thoracic Cavity

Removal of the wall of the thorax reveals abnormal contents such as chylothorax, hydrothorax, pleural exudates and foreign fluids such as milk in the thoracic cavity. Other grossly visible lesions include mediastinal masses, enlarged pericardial sacs due to either effusions or enlarged hearts, and abnormal thoracic contents such as liver and intestine subsequent to a diaphragmatic hernia. Photographs of such lesions are easy to take in small animals which can be positioned under the vertically mounted camera in the photography room. Necropsy technique must be neat, and jagged transected ribs, loose tags of tissue muscle or fat, or extraneous blood on organs or mixed with pleural contents should be avoided. Because modeling is important, either one modeling light alone or with reduced fill-in lighting is required, particularly if the texture of fibrinous exudates (e.g. in fibrinous pleurisy) is to be retained. Cutting the diaphragm as close to its costal attachments as possible reduces the chances of cutting through the site of a diaphragmatic hernia. It also allows the diaphragm to be removed and photographed in its entirety to reveal lesions such as a hernia.

Urinary System

After removal of the lateral wall of the pelvis (Fig. 4.24) (see "Reproductive System"), the urinary system consisting of kidneys, ureters, bladder (including the prostate in males) and urethra is removed *en bloc*, along with the reproductive tract. Where extensive renal infarcts are present, the abdominal aorta and renal arteries should be included in this block and, after removal from the body, the vessels should be opened to reveal any emboli (Ludwig, 1979b). In photographs of the whole urinary system, organs should be arranged vertically as in Figure 4.46. The convention is to view the ventral surface, and thus the left kidney will be on the right.

Kidneys

Preparation. Photographs of individual kidneys are not difficult to take, but the preparation of specimens must be meticulous in order to avoid artefacts. Each kidney should be sliced longitudinally from the greater curvature completely through to the hilus so that both halves are fully separated. This is made easy if the prosector keeps a firm grip on the kidney between thumb and index finger or alternatively lays the kidney flat on a table. If the cut does not separate the two halves completely, parenchyma tends to tear at the point of attachment resulting in an unattractive, ragged surface. As with the brain (Fig. 4.20), liver and lungs, kidneys should be cut with a long straight-bladed knife, using one stroke without to-and-fro motions which may cause serrations or "hesitation" marks on the cut surface. The capsule should be stripped on one-half to reveal the external surface of the kidney and also to demonstrate that there are, or are not, adhesions.

Orientation. Although kidneys lie horizontally in domestic animals,

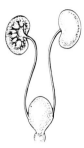

Figure 4.46.

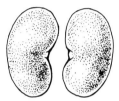

Figure 4.47. Correct anatomic position for viewing the dorsal and ventral surfaces of kidneys. Cranial poles are at the top of the frame.

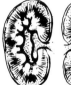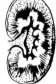

Figure 4.48.

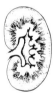

Figure 4.49.

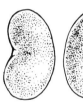

Figure 4.50. Incorrect position of kidney. The hilus should not face towards the outside of the frame but towards the midline as in Figure 4.47.

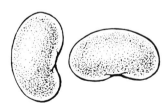

Figure 4.51. Incorrect position of right kidney. The cranial poles should be towards the top of the frame.

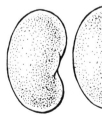

Figure 4.52. Incorrect position of kidney. This position can only be obtained by viewing a dorsal surface of one kidney and a ventral of the other.

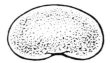

Figure 4.53. Incorrect anatomic
positions of kidney. The cranial
and caudal poles cannot be identified. A horizontal format should
be used only when photographing the lateral surface of quadruped kidneys, not a dorsal or ventral surface.

when the ventral and dorsal surfaces of kidneys, whole or bisected, are
viewed, they should be positioned vertically, with the cranial pole towards
the top of the frame (Figs. 4.47, 4.48, 4.49) (see "Orientation"). Kidneys of
quadrupeds are sometimes placed in a horizontal format (Fig. 4.53). This
is anatomically acceptable only if the lateral or medial surface of the
kidney is viewed—a position rarely used except for bovine kidneys. If
kidneys are placed horizontally, the cranial and caudal poles cannot be
easily identified and, in contrast to vertically oriented kidneys, the
location of lesions cannot be ascertained. Correct orientation of kidneys
avoids the confusing and aesthetically unpleasant arrangements depicted
in Figures 4.50, 4.51 and 4.52. None of these arrangements are possible if
kidneys are correctly oriented and can only be done by either reversing
left and right kidneys or rotating cranial and caudal poles.

    If two whole or two halved kidneys are included in one photograph, a
horizontal format (Figs. 4.47, 4.48) should be used. Like the inclusion of
several slices of any organ (e.g. brain), more than half of the same kidney
merely divides the viewer's attention and should be avoided unless the
two halves are necessary to show the extent or location of a lesion. For
the same reason, if both bisected kidneys are to be photographed, only
half or each and not a total of 4 halves should be included. In kidneys
with glomerulonephritis, pyelonephritis, multiple abscesses, infarcts and
neoplasms, it is advantageous to show both an external and a cut surface
of halved kidneys in one photograph (Halsman and Ishak, 1977). One
half will show the capsular surface and the other a cut surface. Thus, the
kidneys should appear as in Figure 4.54 with the cranial poles at the top
of the frame. Two halves from one kidney can be arranged as in Figure

4.55, only by rotating one half so that its caudal pole is at the top of the frame, thus confusing the viewer.

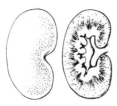

Figure 4.54. Correct anatomic position of the capsular and cut surfaces of two halves of a single sliced kidney. The cranial poles are at the top of the frame.

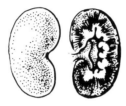

Figure 4.55. Incorrect anatomic position of single sliced kidney. The only way to achieve this arrangement is by rotating one halved kidney so that its cranial pole is toward the bottom of the frame. This misleads the viewer.

Specular Highlights. The cut surfaces of a kidney are often not easy to photograph. If the kidney is flaccid, the cut surface, instead of remaining flat, may curve downward at each pole and one pole may be in shadow. Unfortunately, the curved surface is also prone to produce specular highlights. Both of these problems may be overcome by tilting the background to expose the whole surface of the kidney to light or by propping the specimen up with modeling clay. Tilting the background is easier. Specular highlights can be numerous on the cut surface and cause a serious problem, particularly if kidneys are edematous or have been washed in water or Jores' solution. The use of one light will reduce the number of specular highlights. Left and right lights should be tried independently to see which illumination is the more effective. Also, the specimen and its background should be rotated around the lens axis to select the position at which specular highlights are at a minimum. If all of these procedures are unsatisfactory in reducing specular highlights, polarized lights or even immersion photography, particularly for formalin-fixed material, may be necessary. This has been described under "Lighting" and "Specular Highlights." For very small pieces of fresh kidney, the technique of Burry and Stewart (1973) of supporting small pieces of kidney on the underside of a glass plate can be tried (see "Specular Highlights"). Close-up photographs of either fixed or fresh kidney are frequently plagued with such highlights, as light is reflected from glomeruli with amyloid or from the convoluted tubules of the nephron.

Ureters

Visible lesions include those in which there is a change in shape and/or size, e.g. distension with urine (in hydroureter), pus (pyelitis) or calculi or absence as in atresia. Differences in diameter of a ureter are often best demonstrated by photographing kidneys and ureters *in situ*, usually after the removal of intestines so that ureters are visible. After photography, the urinary system should be removed, photographed *en bloc* and then ureters dilated by pus opened with fine iris scissors to reveal the nature of the exudate.

Renal Vessels

Obstruction of a renal artery by a thrombus or embolus is rare in domestic animals, but such lesions should be demonstrated either with the kidney *in situ* or after removal of the urinary system, aorta and renal vessels *en bloc*. The embolus is demonstrated by opening along the length of the aorta and renal vessels (Ludwig, 1979b).

Urinary Bladder and Urethra

When the urinary system is removed *en bloc*, the urethra remains attached to the urinary bladder. The female urethra and bladder should be opened by a dorsal midline incision starting at the urethral orifice after the vagina has been opened by a dorsal midsagittal incision. In man, the urethra is opened in the anterior (ventral) midline (Ludwig, 1979b). Because the penile urethra of male domestic animals is surrounded dorsally and laterally by a corpus cavernosum (and in the case of the dog, by a bone), the only site at which the urethra is readily accessible is by a midventral incision. The penis of many domestic animals is horizontal, and consequently this incision corresponds to a posterior (dorsal) incision in man and primates. At the ischial arch, the urethra makes a U-shaped change in direction and the ventral incision becomes a dorsal one and should be continued in the midsagittal plane along the dorsal surface of the urinary bladder. In this way the trigone is preserved and the bladder lumen revealed. Many animals die with the urinary bladder contracted and at necropsy the walls may appear thickened and turgid. However, after a middorsal incision, the walls can usually be spread apart to reveal the lumen and contents. If the walls are stiff and will not reflect, a portion of the dorsal wall may be excised in a fashion similar to that described for the trachea (see "Respiratory System"). Contents such as calculi can then be photographed *in situ.* For photography, the long axis of the bladder should be oriented vertically, because its dorsal surface is being viewed. The cranial pole (fundus) should be at the top of the frame (Fig. 4.56) and never in the reverse direction.

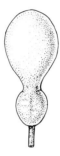

Figure 4.56.

In some cases the bladder should be fixed distended. Urine should be withdrawn by catheter and then fixatives such as 10% NBF gently infused to distend the bladder (Ludwig, 1979b). This procedure is most useful if it is desired to slice the bladder into serial transverse sections, a technique useful to demonstrate location and extent of lesions. This technique has been used to depict the sequence of re-epithelialization of the urinary bladder from the trigone after the mucosa has been stripped surgically. Serial sections should be oriented in correct sequence with the most cranial slice at the top of the frame, dorsal surface of the bladder towards the top and the left side of the bladder to the left of the frame. These recommendations are similar to those for brain slices, discussed under "Nervous System."

Photographs of traumatized urinary bladders with rupture, avulsion or retroperitoneal hemorrhage may be more convincing if photographed with the urinary system *in situ,* after removal of the lateral wall of the pelvis (see "Pelvic Cavity" under "Abdominal Cavity.")

Penis

The penis may not be visible until the prepuce has been incised, most conveniently done by a ventral midline incision (i.e. immediately ventral to the incision to be made into the penile urethra). Photographs of the external penis are usually made to record lesions such as squamous cell carcinoma in horses, transmissible venereal tumor in dogs or calculi in the urethral process of sheep. During life, the normal orientation of the long axis of the penis varies from species to species, but it is approximately horizontal in most domestic animals except the cat and primates. Thus, in photographs of a lateral surface, the penis of most domestic animals should be oriented horizontally (Fig. 4.57). In dorsal and ventral view of the penises of all animals and lateral views of primates, the penis should be positioned with its long axis vertical. The glans may be directed towards the bottom or top of the frame (Fig. 4.57). The latter is a better position for photography under the standardized lights.

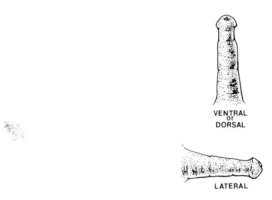

VENTRAL
or
DORSAL

LATERAL

Figure 4.57. In dorsal and ventral views of the penises of quadrupeds, the penis should be vertical. In views of a lateral surface, the penis should be horizontal.

CADAVER PHOTOGRAPHY

Photography of two types of subject is discussed here: (a) intact bodies and (b) organs *in situ* in the dissected body. Photography of *in situ* organs in human and large animal cadavers is difficult, but the bodies of laboratory animals and small animals weighing less than 70 pounds can be carried to a photography room and photographed under the vertically mounted camera. The latter technique results in photographs of excellent quality and facilitates recording sequential dissections of organs *in situ.* Necropsy technique must be meticulous with neatly transected ribs, tags of tissues removed and no contamination of organs by blood and feces. As Pilcher (1937) points out, a series of photographs to show the progressive dissection of lesions is invaluable and cannot be duplicated later once the organs have been removed from the body. Also, in our experience, the prosector cannot always tell the stage of dissection at which lesions are demonstrated optimally for photography. Thus, it is easy to dissect too far and, for example, puncture and deflate a cyst or emphysematous bulla.

Preparation of the Intact Cadaver for Photography

Exactly what preparation will be done depends on the purpose of the photograph. To document the appearance of legal cases at the time of death, no preparation is required or desired. However, once these photographs have been taken, aesthetic changes should be made. These include removal of bandages, splints, intravenous drips and identification labels or collars. Blood stains may be removed by washing with physiological saline. Large animals coated with mud or bedding should be washed down to reveal skin lesions such as abrasions, lacerations or self-inflicted injuries such as those frequently seen on the head of horses with colic. Feces on the peritoneum in a case of diarrhea should be photographed before being washed off.

Large Animal Cadaver Photography

Photographs of whole bodies of animals, particularly large animals, are difficult to take and their use is frequently limited to legal and insurance cases or to show the position at the time of death. For example, horses with hepatic encephalopathy may walk into the fork of a tree and die there. In general, bodies should be photographed immediately after death. Cadavers stored in a refrigerator, whether they have been placed in plastic sacks or not, may have wet matted hair, or the body may be distorted by rigor mortis into unrealistic and unattractive positions.

A transilluminated background can be used for small bodies and an opaque background such as laminated plastic can be used for larger cadavers. The major difficulties in large animal cadaver photography are discussed under the following headings:

- Lighting
- Background

• Perspective, Viewpoint and Orientation

Lighting. Necropsy room floors and tables are often wet and may be contaminated. Thus, because of the danger of electrocution to the photographer and contamination of equipment, the use of cameras on tripods and floodlights on stands with electric cables is contraindicated. The danger of electrocution from cables on wet floors is reduced by using retractable spools mounted on the ceiling. However, even these cables will inevitably become contaminated. Frequently, there are only two safe alternatives, either available light or electronic flash.

Available Light. The type of lighting in the necropsy room will dictate whether or not it is suitable for photography. For example, a mixture of lights of different color temperatures (e.g. skylight and tungsten light) cannot be balanced for use with color film. Kodak (1984) published recommendations for color-compensating (CC) filters for a variety of fluorescent tubes and high-intensity discharge lamps. Our necropsy room is brightly illuminated (100 ft. candles on the benchtops) by high-intensity mercury lamps (deluxe white) which produce an overall greenish cast on film. However, by using color-compensating filters (CC40M + CC10Y) over the camera's lens, the result is a good but not a faithful record of the colors on Ektachrome 200. However, even with this high level of illumination, exposures with a fast film (Ektachrome 200) are still relatively long, 1/60 second at f-4. Thus, depth of field is inadequate for hand-held close-up photographs, and tripods must be used to allow longer exposure times and small apertures. The equivalent exposure time is ¼ second at f-16. Kodak (1983) states that reciprocity failure does not occur with this film until exposures are as long as 1 second, and even then this does not produce a color cast. To obtain a suitable viewpoint, tripods should be adjustable up to 6 feet in height. To prevent the spread of infection out of the necropsy laboratory, a tripod should be kept for exclusive use in the necropsy room. Also, a mobile platform may be necessary to elevate the photographer to enable him to look through the viewfinder of the camera.

Electronic Flash for Large Animal Cadaver Photography. The other alternative is to use electronic flash. Over the years the results have been adequate but not excellent because of the inability to have a hand-held camera fitted with two flash units—one as a main light and the other on the camera as fill-in illumination. Results have been highly variable, and even if exposure were correct, often lighting was flat and texture and modeling poor. This situation has changed recently. Now excellent flash photographs with modeling (Fig. 4.58) and fill-in illumination and automatic exposure control with excellent repeatability are possible because of small dedicated flash units with exposure controlled by meters reading directly off the film plane (TTL–OTF). This new technique has changed the whole approach to cadaver photography. The equipment has been described under "Equipment" and techniques under "Skin and Special Senses."

Plus X Pan film developed in D-76 (1 + 1) for the times given in Table XIII have produced excellent results. The development times are based on those recommended by Kodak (1984b) to give a contrast index of 0.42 recommended for negatives to be enlarged on a condensor enlarger—the type usually used with 35mm negatives. However, because electronic flash units with exposures of less than 1/1000 second cause reciprocity failure, Kodak recommends a 10%–15% increase in development time (Table XIII).

If there is good color contrast between lesions and normal tissue, flash photography with a single-flash unit can produce reasonably good results. An example is pneumonic lung with grey consolidated lobules and pink normal lobules. But flash photographs can be disappointing because of lack of modeling from flat lighting, reflections from glossy surfaces and uneven illumination. These defects are likely to occur if a single-flash unit is used on the camera and the field of view is large, as for example the opened abdomen of a horse. Even illumination with a single, laterally placed flash unit is easiest to obtain with relatively small fields of view, about 12 × 18 inches to 6 × 9 inches (RR = 1:12 to RR = 1:6 with 35mm cameras). The lateral position of the flash produces some modeling.

In photographing large animal cadavers, several views such as a "long shot" for orientation and a "close-up" photograph for detail may be required. This is common practice in veterinary clinical photography (Fritts, 1976). The problem in taking photographs of large animals is to include sufficient anatomic landmarks to orient the viewer and, at the same time, to keep lesions sufficiently large to show detail. Frequently, the only answer is to take two or more photographs. Sometimes with large animals it may be possible to record detail and orient the viewer in the one photograph. For example, if a steer with Stephanofilarial dermatitis of the peri-umbilical skin is placed in lateral recumbency and photographed from a point caudal and ventrolateral to the umbilicus

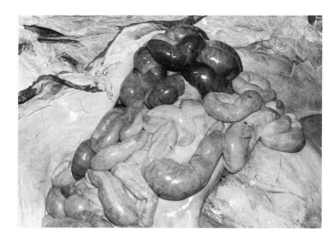

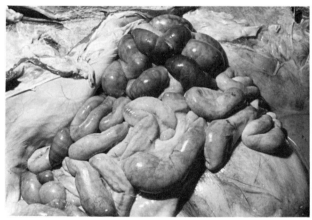

Figure 4.58. Comparison of modeling in photographs of viscera of a cadaver in lateral recumbency taken with (*top*) single flash unit mounted on the camera and (*lower*) twin dedicated flash units with the modeling light held by an assistant above and to the left and with the fill-in flash unit at ⅛th output mounted on the camera. Exposure was controlled automatically by the TTL–OTF metering of the camera. (*lower*) Notice that modeling is excellent.

and in a cranio-dorsal direction, the photograph will include the lesion, a ventrolateral view of the thorax and neck, and even portions of the head. The latter will act as landmarks which will aid in orientation of the viewer.

As the working distance increases, illumination from the flash mounted close to the camera will become flat and provide little indication of texture or modeling in the photograph. Therefore, it is even more important to have an assistant hold the flash head at a 30°–50° elevation

Table XIII
TIME-TEMPERATURE TABLE FOR PLUS X PAN FILM
DEVELOPED IN D-76 DILUTED 1 + 1,
IN SMALL TANK INVERTED EVERY 30 SECONDS.

Temperature °F	Contrast Index CI = 0.42	10% Increase For Flash Photography
65	5 min. 10 sec.	5 min. 40 sec.
68	4 min. 30 sec.	5 min.
70	4 min. 10 sec.	4 min. 35 sec.
72	3 min. 50 sec.	4 min. 10 sec.
75	3 min. 10 sec.	3 min. 30 sec.

Development times at the different temperatures are the same percentage of change as listed for D-76 (1 +1) reported in Kodak Bulletin AJ-16, 1984.

above and to the side of the camera's optical axis. The modeling light flash unit should be directed into an orifice. For example, when photographing an opened oral cavity of a head lying on its left side and facing to the right, the flash would be held on the right side of the camera and directed into the mouth. Fritts (1976) explains that "this prevents the bridge of the nose from interfering with the lighting and also tends to throw any shadows behind the lesion." If the flash head is mounted on the other side of the camera, not only is the depth of the oral cavity not illuminated, but a large distracting shadow is present rostral to the mouth.

Background. Backgrounds are extremely difficult to control in the photography of large animal cadavers. Clutter from stainless steel tables, tile and terrazzo floors and multiple obtrusive horizontal and vertical lines as well as blood and feces are a problem. Also, if the angle of view is low, distracting objects in the background will be clearly visible. This problem also exists in the photography of human cadavers (Smialowski and Currie, 1960a). To minimize the amount of background and prevent distortion, the camera's optical axis should be at 90° to the surface photographed (Fig. 4.59). This usually requires a high viewpoint and either the hydraulic necropsy table can be lowered, a short stepladder used or both. If the working distance of the lens is increased by using a lens with a longer focal length (e.g. 105mm instead of the "standard" 50mm on a 35mm camera), the angle subtended by the subject is reduced and less background is included in the photograph. Another alternative is to use a 40mm–105mm zoom lens to select the field with the minimum amount of background.

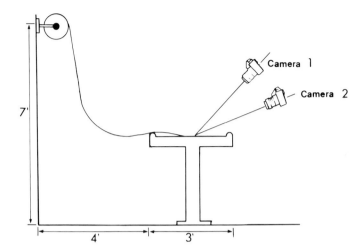

Figure 4.59. The camera's optical axis should be at approximately 90° to the surface of the subject (camera 1). This prevents distortion, minimizes the depth of the subject so that it remains within the depth of field, and reduces or eliminates extraneous background which is greater at camera 2 position.

We use black plastic laminated boards as backgrounds. These are very successful under small animal cadavers or behind portions, such as the head of large animal cadavers. Stainless steel is totally unsuitable as a background, as it can record in photographs either as a bright gleaming surface or as a dark grey. If the cadaver is on a stainless steel table, alternative backgrounds are black plastic laminate-covered boards (see "Equipment") or pull-down vinyl or disposable paper backgrounds (Fig. 4.59). These are not popular, as they are difficult to keep clean but in some cases may be the lesser of the evils. Our floor is light grey with a reflectance of approximately 40 percent. If the floor is used as a background, care should be taken to insure that defects such as cracks in the paint or floor drains are not visible. Care must be taken to be sure that light sources from the flash or overhead lamps are not reflected by the light grey background into the camera lens, as this causes gleaming specular highlights.

All extraneous material should be removed. Blood and exudate may have to be blotted away repeatedly. The floor or table should be cleared of all debris and blood. For monochrome photography, every attempt should be made to include a ruler at the very edge of the frame. Later, this can be cropped off and size indicated by a line drawn by an artist (see "Ruler").

Perspective, Viewpoint and Orientation

It is important to remember to orient the cadaver in its anatomically correct position. Correct orientation depends on two factors: whether the animal is a quadruped or a biped and whether the pleural and peritoneal cavities have been opened from the lateral or ventral approach. Quadruped animals are usually necropsied in lateral recumbency, and the upper abdominal and thoracic walls are reflected to reveal viscera. Thus, quadrupeds should be photographed in a horizontal format with their dorsal surface towards the top of frame. Bipeds such as monkeys and birds and all quadrupeds autopsied in dorsal recumbency, and thus with the thoracic and abdominal cavities opened from a ventral approach, should be positioned in a vertical format with the head towards the top of the frame. In both cases, light should come from the top or top left.

The rule most often ignored is to have the camera's optical axis at 90° to the plane to be photographed. The usual fault is too low a viewpoint which can cause distortion of that portion of the body nearest the camera and result in the inclusion of an excessive amount of background. A step stool or stepladder is frequently required to allow the photographer to photograph a complete body cavity in a large animal (Fritts, 1976).

Monochrome Photographs of Lesions *in Situ* in the Necropsy Room

Good results have been obtained with diffused room light from high-intensity mercury lamps mounted 20 feet above the floor. The lighting is shadowless, diffuse, but still directional. White walls give adequate fill-in illumination. The camera must be tripod mounted or clamped to a small stepladder. Fast films such as Kodak Tri-X (400 ISO) have given excellent tonal gradation and resolution when used with high-quality lenses. Six by eight inch enlargements which are more than large enough for publication are of satisfactory quality. Any distracting background can be masked off in the print. However, the twin dedicated flash units have superceded available light photography. Excellent results have been obtained using Kodak Plus X Pan film (Fig. 4.58). The selection of this film was based on the necessity of using a film with sufficient "speed" to allow the use of apertures such as f-11 and f-16 with the dedicated flash unit. Details of development are given above under "Lighting."

Chapter 5

CLINICAL PHOTOGRAPHY

Photographs to illustrate lesions or clinical signs in live animals should really be portraits. Good clinical photographs are very difficult to take. When one considers the equipment, lighting, space and cooperation, to say nothing of the photographer's skill required to make good clinical photographs of human patients (Kodak, 1972a), the problems in photographing uncooperative animals seem enormous. Thus, the photography of animal patients has much in common with the photography of pediatric patients, and the statement that success or failure [of pediatric photography] depends to a great extent on the attitude of the patient, the help of the mother, and the ingenuity of the photographer; good luck also plays an important role! applies also to veterinary medicine. Taking clinical photographs of animals frequently becomes an attempt to eliminate the most glaring faults by choosing the least objectionable background, obtain sufficient light to give adequate depth of field and "freeze" subject motion. These requirements frequently preclude any option to choose the direction or type of lighting, the factors which are most important in illuminating the lesion optimally.

To take excellent photographs of live animals requires the following:

1. flexible lighting whose direction can be adjusted in accordance with the nature of the lesion. Thus, texture lighting is required to record the surface of granulating ulcers and rim lighting to emphasize the outline of distorted limbs. The light should be of sufficient intensity to allow the use of small lens apertures to provide adequate depth of field to ensure that the whole subject is in focus and exposures short enough to "freeze" subject and camera motion. Lighting should also be dependable and safe, and these requirements are essentially the same as those for human pediatric photography (Rogers, 1976).
2. An unobtrusive background.

247

Purpose of Clinical Photographs

Appreciation of the difficulties of lighting clinical subjects is made easier if the objectives for taking these photographs are understood. These can be categorized as follows:

1. **Location of Lesions.** Examples are photodynamic dermatitis affecting the unpigmented areas of a body, distribution of gunshot wounds and anatomic location of tumors. In these photographs, there is relatively little fine detail. Diffused, even lighting to prevent deep shadows and a plain unobtrusive background are the major requirements.

2. **Change in Shape or Contour.** When there are changes in external contour such as those due to arthrogryposis, lordosis or kyphosis, change in outline can be accentuated by the use of modeling or rim lighting combined with a contrasting background. Even if optimal lighting is not available, a diffuse, relatively even illumination will be adequate if the background contrasts strongly with the outline of the animal. Obviously, a single color or grey tone will not provide a suitably contrasting background for all animals. A light background is required for dark animals and vice versa. Thus, a variety of backgrounds are needed. More subtle changes in contour, such as those due to atrophy of muscle groups, are difficult to photograph successfully. In human subjects, this is done by using modeling lights to illuminate the contours and with the subject cooperating in positioning and tensing muscles. Above all, the services of a highly skilled photographer are required. Frontal lighting, particularly from numerous light sources positioned near the camera, is usually unsuitable to show changes in outline or posture. Multiple lights cast multiple shadows of legs which confuse and mask the outline of the body. Shadows on the background can only be prevented by having sufficient distance between the animal and the background, by additional background lighting or by using a completely diffused light to illuminate subject and background. Good photographs of deformed limbs of horses have been taken with backlighting from the sun which has essentially produced "rim" lighting, i.e. light on the outside of the legs against a dark background. To obtain such results, the sunlight must be at a low angle and the background uniformly dark.

3. **Change in Posture or Gait.** These may be due to a neurological deficit, behavioral change or some mechanical defect. Typical examples are ataxia from cerebellar hypoplasia, dysmetria from degeneration of

the dorsal funiculus in pigs with organophosphate poisoning, sagging of facial muscles and/or ear from facial paralysis, circling in ovine listerosis and limberneck in birds with botulism. Behavioral changes include head pressing in horses with hepatic encephalopathy, "star gazing" in chickens with nutritional encephalomalacia (vitamin E deficiency) and opisthotonos caused by tetanus and strychnine poisoning. Mechanical defects such as overgrown horns, chronic laminitis and contracted tendons change the posture of horses. Photographs to show changes in posture and gait require relatively even illumination (to prevent deep shadows) combined with a plain contrasting background. Diffuse sunlight is probably the easiest to use. A long plain concrete wall and apron (Fig. 5.1) preferably with the wall-floor junction coved to eliminate a horizontal line is good. Other alternative backgrounds such as only a concrete or asphalt apron, grass (Fig. 5.2), or pasture (Fig. 5.3) should be used with a high viewpoint to minimize the extent of the background.

4. **Details in External Lesions.** These should accurately depict color and texture in skin lesions. With large animals, it is rare to be able to record good detail and also show the anatomic location in one photograph. Two photographs may be required, one to include the whole or most of the body to show location and the other to reveal the lesion in a close-up. Diffused even lighting required for the former is unsuitable for the latter for which modeling or texture lighting is essential. The camera with the twin dedicated flash units described in "Equipment" is suitable, as it gives modeling with relatively even illumination. An unobtrusive background is required.

Photographic Equipment

For most photography, a 35mm single-lens-reflex camera is excellent. However, lenses with focal lengths longer than the so-called normal 55mm lens are desirable. The longer focal length means that the angle subtended by the lens is less, and thus to cover the same field of view, the camera's viewpoint has to be moved further back. Thus, the lens-subject (working) distance is increased. This "flattens" the perspective which is another way of saying that distortion due to some parts of the body being closer to the lens than others is reduced. Also, what is more significant is that the photographer distracts the animal less and also the photographer is safer. For clinical photography, lenses of 85mm–105mm and sometimes 135mm focal lengths are used. The 105mm lens is excellent

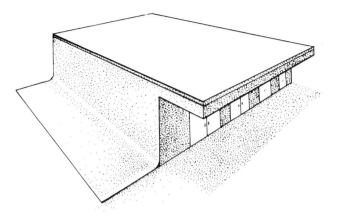

Figure 5.1. Outdoor background for large animal photography. The south-facing wall of a large animal examination room has been converted into a seamless background by plastering the wall and coving it to the concrete apron.

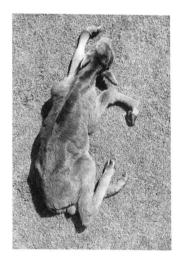

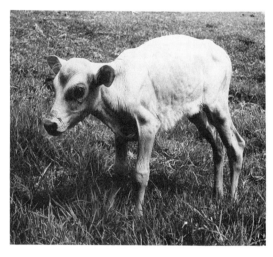

Figure 5.2. (*Left*) Lawn background. The texture of the closely cropped grass is obtrusive.

Figure 5.3. (*Right*) Pasture background. A high viewpoint and the use of a long focal length lens has kept the background relatively simple. Courtesy of G. I. Alexander.

for photographs of small animals, as the perspective is pleasing and the animals are not distracted by the photographer, but the working distance of the lens is still close enough to allow the use of small apertures with electronic flash units of moderate output. Zoom lenses (50mm–135mm focal length) should be ideal for clinical photography, but in 1976, Rogers (1976) found that they were not as good optically as fixed focal length lenses. Zoom lenses have improved, but it may be desirable to test them before using them routinely.

Rogers (1976) also advocates the use of a larger format camera for black-and-white photography. He uses a 6cm × 6cm camera for two reasons:

1. "a far greater amount of precision and care in handling is necessary with 35mm film in order to achieve good quality prints without marks or blemishes since the skill of assistance vary, . . . this precision is not always guaranteed."
2. The viewfinder image of a 6 × 6 camera is of sufficient size to allow accurate positioning of the subject within the negative area.

If relatively little black-and-white photography is done, the cost of a larger format camera is probably not justified. Another point to remember is that the depth of field with the larger format is less because the image is larger and thus the RR is closer to 1:1. If depth of field is barely adequate with the flash-film combination for a 35mm camera, it will be inadequate with the larger format, and higher output electronic flash units may be required.

Backgrounds

Judged by the slides presented at professional meetings, backgrounds are a major problem in both small-animal and large-animal photography. Fritts (1976) considers that background distractions are the most difficult problems in photography of large animals. This is because of the structures used to restrain animals, particularly large unbroken animals. As Fritts (1976) points out, "restraining devices [for large animals] are designed for efficient use by the veterinarian with no thought given to the photographer's problems." Thus, in the case of unbroken animals, there may be no alternative but to photograph them in a chute. The only option the photographer has is to try to minimize the background by framing and composition. However for animals which are more amenable to handling, some of the backgrounds discussed below can be used. With advanced planning, a plain wall can be incorporated during construction into the restraining area for unbroken animals.

The discussion on backgrounds under "Gross Pathological Specimens" emphasized that backgrounds should be unobtrusive and may or may not accentuate the outline of the subject. Desirable features in a background in clinical photographs are:

1. **Plain, Homogeneous.** This implies the absence of horizontal or vertical lines at wall-to-wall or wall-to-floor junctions. Poor backgrounds are extremely common in photographs of large animals. Defects include horizontal lines from doorway frames, edges of road, horizontal air-intake grills, roof lines, power lines, corral fences, patches in the blacktop, weeds between blacktop and white barn wall, horizontal mortar lines in brick walls (Fig. 5.4), and "no parking" signs. Vertical lines have resulted from the inclusion of utility poles, tree trunks, pole barns, smokestacks, vertically corrugated iron walls, shadows of legs of horse, down-pipes, vertical expansion joints in brick walls, vertical phone lines on barn walls, and isolated legs of an animal holder whose body was obscured by the body of a horse. Changes in background texture or color are caused by patched or cracked blacktop, and patches of snow or dirt on blacktop or concrete.

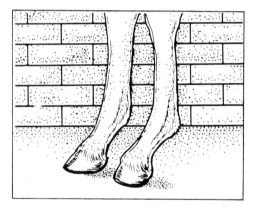

Figure 5.4. Brick wall background. The mortar lines are obtrusive and distracting. The wall should be plastered and coved to the floor as in Figure 5.1.

One defect in backgrounds which can usually be controlled is clutter. This includes the presence of such items as garbage cans, automobiles, vans with labels, animal feces, hoses and animal handlers. The eye is unerringly drawn to people, automobiles and lettering such as "no parking" signs and identification badges. The distraction caused by automobiles is so complete that many viewers will attempt to identify type, model and year and completely ignore the intended subject. Animal handlers are photographic "clutter" and can be very distracting (Fig. 5.5), particularly if they are attractive. Their clothing and haircuts are examined for style and era and name badges are read. If possible, the photographer should attempt to exclude handlers. This can be done if the animal will remain in place without any restraint or if it is held on a long halter rope with the handler out of the photograph. While the rope will lead the eye out of the photograph, it is still less distracting than including parts of the hands and body of a handler. However, the halter and ropes must be inconspicuous—not brightly colored or multicolored. If handlers must be included, they should be made as inconspicuous as possible by wearing olive drab coveralls, a surgeon's cap to cover red or blonde hair, and gloves to prevent their manicure from being inspected in close-up photographs. Their hands should be kept as far from the animal as possible and should not touch the animal so that the portion of the handler unavoidably visible in the photograph can be masked off in a print or transparency.

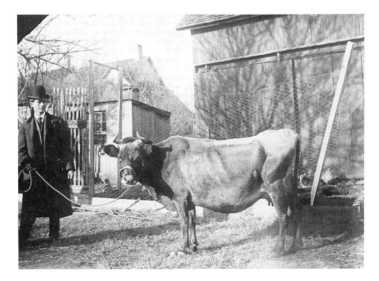

Figure 5.5. Historical photograph of a tuberculous cow. Because of the age of the photograph, the background is now more interesting than the subject. Courtesy, Dean, College of Veterinary Medicine, Kansas State University.

2. **Colored, Black, Grey or White.** In the 1950s, blue-green was advocated as a background color by Gibson (1950) and Harris (1956), and green and blue backgrounds are still used today. Later, Kodak (1972a) recommended that the background and floor be "painted a light aqua blue-green diluted with white." This color selection was based on the assumption that as red and yellow hues predominate in human skins, a complementary background color was desirable to "enhance the color." The distortion of the perception of color by colored backgrounds has been discussed under "Backgrounds." For the correct appreciation of colors, backgrounds should be neutral (i.e. grey, black or white). Even if colored backgrounds were desirable, there is no justification for using a blue-green for all animals when coat colors vary from black, brown, red to white. Another disadvantage of colored backgrounds is that shadows cast on them change not only in tone (grey scale value) but also in color saturation. Thus, changes in colored backgrounds are very obvious, particularly when caused by multiple complex shadows. If the use of colored backgrounds is eliminated, the alternatives are white, grey and black. Rogers (1976) found grey backgrounds had two serious problems in photography of children. He found it impossible to maintain the same grey tone in prints from the one case over a period. Also, contrast between the grey background and caucasian skin was insufficient. For this reason he standardized on white backgrounds for photographic prints. The problem of variability in the tone of grey backgrounds also applies to photography of animals. The second problem of the lack of contrast between subject and light grey background is less likely to occur with domestic animals because many have dark coats. Thus, light grey backgrounds are frequently the best compromise in veterinary medicine for both color transparencies and black-and-white prints.

Functional Backgrounds for Large Animals

Alternatives are:

1. **Portrait Studios.** A completely equipped studio with interchangeable backgrounds and flexible studio lighting is a rarity for large animals. Kodak's (1972a) recommendation is that for human patient photography, the area should be at least 12 × 16 ft. and preferably 16 × 20 ft., with a minimum 9 ft. ceiling. Obviously, large domestic animals require more space than humans. The Ohio State University College of Veterinary Medicine has such a studio.

2. **Plain Concrete Wall and Apron.** These should be completely plain

and free of grills, doors, windows, cabinets, switches, electrical outlets and expansion joints between concrete slabs. They can be outside (Fig. 5.1) or inside the building. An outside wall should run approximately east-west, and face south in the northern hemisphere in order to be illuminated by sunlight or overcast sky for most of the year. The junction between the wall and the floor should be coved with at least a 1 ft. and preferably a 2 ft. radius so that there is no sharp horizontal line between background and floor. The wall should be a minimum of 10 ft. and preferably 12 to 15 ft. high so that the background will be adequate to photograph the head of a horse from a low angle. Although 15 ft. is an adequate length of background for many large animals in full side view, a 60 to 100 ft. wall allows oblique views and the wall can also be used for motion pictures or television recording of the gait of animals. A length of 60 ft. should be considered minimal. Eighty feet is good and 100 ft. excellent. Many large animal hospitals have outside walls or inside walls 100 to 150 ft. long. The concrete apron against the wall should be a minimum of 12 ft. and preferably 16 ft. deep to allow sufficient space for the animal to stand away from the wall and thus prevent hard shadows being cast on the background or to allow the background to be illuminated separately. Kodak (1972) recommends a minimum of a 6 ft. wide floor for human patients. The concrete apron should be swept clean before each photographic session. In the absence of a concrete wall, a high viewpoint and a plain concrete slab may be adequate for photography of small subjects and feet of large animals. Suitable inside walls are frequently present in the corridors of large animal veterinary hospitals. Our hospital has a wall 15 ft. high × 150 ft. long, but air-conditioning ducts have reduced the useful height to 12 ft. and the floor drains are located against the wall and are distracting. With preliminary planning, the full 15 ft. high wall could have been made into a suitable background. Another possibility is to use a wall of a large animal treatment room (Fig. 5.6). With preplanning, one wall could be kept completely free of power outlets, switches, air conditioning ducts, water and drain pipes. These examination rooms are frequently large, and the one at the University of Tennessee Veterinary Teaching Hospital is 50 × 35 × 16 ft. high. At little expense, the 35 ft. long wall could be plastered with concrete and coved to the floor. Another requirement is that there be no floor drains 12 to 16 ft. from the wall. The wall, cove and floor can be painted with light grey epoxy paint with a reflectance of approximately 40 percent. The painted floor will inevitably become damaged by the feet of animals and will require frequent repainting. If the available wall is too short, Kodak (1972) recommends using two adjoining walls by rounding the corners between the walls with a vertical cove of about 3 ft. radius. For human subjects 5–6 ft. of each wall are required (Kodak, 1972).

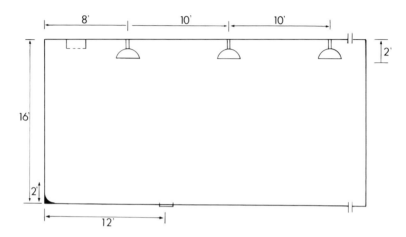

Figure 5.6. Indoor photographic background. Side elevation of interior of the large animal examination room depicted in Figure 5.1. The left wall is plain, devoid of windows, pipes, air ducts, electrical switches and outlets and is coved to the floor which is also plain and has no drains for 12 feet from the wall.

3. **Pull-Down Backgrounds.** Retractable rolls of paper are commercially available. They should be a minimum of 15 ft. wide for large animals such as horses and cattle, but rolls 12 ft. wide have been used. Twelve feet is barely adequate for a large horse in side view. As the paper usually becomes soiled and cannot be reused, paper costs can be very high. If the distance between the camera and the wall is long enough, a long focal length lens can be used, as it has the advantage of not only reducing distortion but also requiring a smaller background. It is desirable that there be space between the background and the animal so that cast shadows, particularly of the legs, fall on the floor and not on the background.

4. **Animals in the Sun and the Background in Deep Shadow.** Occasionally, backgrounds will be required to emphasize changes in the outline such as bowed legs, lordosis, etc. Here a contrasting background is required to attract the eye to the edge of the body. For light-colored animals this can be achieved by photographing them in sunlight at a low angle against the black shadow of a building.

5. **Snow.** Plain non-glaring snow produces a light background suitable for monochrome prints. It is particularly successful in close-ups where the background is out of focus.

6. **Sky.** A clear sky can be a suitable background in color or black and white, but the angle of view which reveals the lesion best may not include sky as a background. Unless the animal is standing on a hill, a low camera angle will be necessary, and even then it may be difficult to avoid having utility wires and buildings visible.

7. **Pasture.** Occasionally, there will be no alternative but to photograph unrestrained animals on pasture. A high camera viewpoint will confine the background to the pasture (Fig. 5.3). Short grass is much to be preferred to long, but a close-cropped lawn will have a distinct and distracting texture (Fig. 5.2). Wherever possible, the subject, rather than the background, should display the more noticeable texture, as a strongly patterned or blotchy background detracts from the subject (Kodak, 1972b).

8. **Backgrounds with Gridlines.** To record growth, animals such as cattle can be photographed against a background covered by gridlines, usually 10cm or 25cm apart (Fig. 5.7). The method is unreliable unless the dorsal line of the animal is level with the optical axis of the camera. If the camera points up or down, the gridlines will be displaced in relation to the animal's dorsal line. To avoid this, a bubble level should be used in the camera's flash shoe to ensure that the optical axis is horizontal. A long-focus lens, such as a 100mm to 135mm on a 35mm camera, will increase the working distance and minimize, but not eliminate, distortion at the edges of the grid. An alternative and probably more accurate method applicable to photographic prints is the one described by Rogers (1976) for pediatric photographs. He photographed a scale on the next frame at exactly the same magnification. This implies that the scale was positioned in the principal plane of focus without refocusing the camera. Later, the scale was printed on the bottom of the print of the patient.

9. **Unsuitable Backgrounds in Publication Prints.** Occasionally, there may be no choice but to take photographs with a completely unsuitable background (Fig. 5.8). This is most likely to happen with unbroken large animals which have to be restrained in a corral or chute. Corral fences and rails are particularly distracting in motion pictures, television and color transparencies. Photographs of animals in chutes are frequently poor and the only alternative left to the photographer is to try to frame the area of interest to minimize the amount of chute visible. In monochrome photographs for publication, an expert photographic depart-

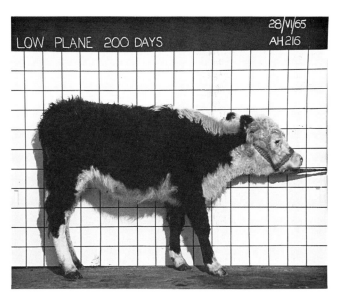

Figure 5.7. Grid background with lines 10cm apart. This type of background can give incorrect measurements unless the camera's optical axis is at the same height as the top line of the animal. A long focal length lens with a long working distance is essential to minimize distortion. Courtesy of Doctor J. G. Morris.

ment can retouch or airbrush the background (Fig. 5.8). Retouching may be done either on the print, the original negative or, if the latter is very small, on a copy negative made from an enlarged print. The easiest method is to paint the background on the print light grey while leaving the foreground untouched. If the foreground is concrete, the background can be painted to match its tone.

No matter which of the alternatives is used, it is obvious from the preceding discussion that backgrounds for large animals need to be planned. Unfortunately, many veterinary institutions have not done this, and distracting backgrounds are frequently seen in photographs, movies and television tapes. The question is, which background to choose? While complete facilities to take portraits are desirable, the cost is very high. For most existing facilities, the decision is which is the least undesirable but still relatively versatile. Backgrounds of snow, sky and pasture are difficult to use and the position of the animal to obtain the best background may not be the one with the best lighting of the subject. The most versatile outdoor background is the concrete wall and apron. If it is large, different viewing angles are possible. Previous discussion has indicated that no one background tone is suitable for animals of all

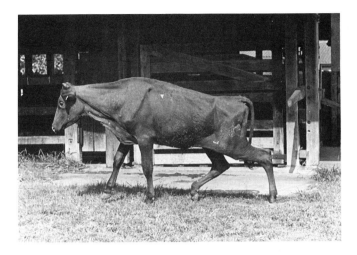

Figure 5.8a. Steer with proprioceptive deficit and dysmetria in front of a cluttered background, unsuitable for publication.

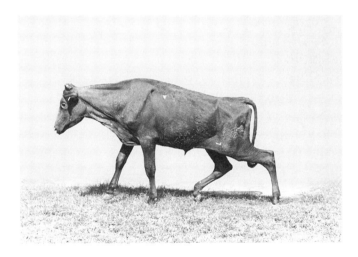

Figure 5.8b. The same photograph with the background airbrushed to a plain grey (McWilliams Photo Retouching, Knoxville, TN 37917).

colors or for all purposes. A compromise has to be made in building such a wall, as it is not possible to change its color or tone. If the concrete remains unblemished and a uniform grey, it may be suitable and economical. However, if there are blotches, changes in color and texture or cracks, the wall and apron will have to be painted a light grey with a reflectance of approximately 40 percent. Preliminary experiments should be made to determine which grey tone is most suitable. Our experience has been that paints which appear neutral grey to the eye may have a distinct color cast towards either green or blue on color films. Therefore, preliminary trials are essential.

Photographic Backgrounds for Small Animal Clinical Photographs

The problems here are basically similar to those with large animals, which is the presence of distracting backgrounds. Outdoor photographs of small animals are likely to be taken from a high viewpoint which reduces the size of the background and the number of distractions. Backgrounds used in indoor photographs have included green surgical towels complete with obvious texture and folds, walls with prominent wall-floor junctions and with cabinets and stainless steel items. Even some planed backgrounds are distracting because of wall-floor lines or heavily saturated colors such as a deep blue which has the additional disadvantage of reflecting blue light over the subject. With planning, a suitable background can be established at a relatively low cost. An immediately available background greatly facilitates photography.

Backgrounds and light-subject distances are smaller and allow the use of lower output artificial light sources, thus reducing costs. Most still photographs can be taken indoors with artificial light.

Choices of backgrounds include:

1. **Portrait Studios.** The one that has been described for large animals is also suitable for small animals. Animals which are not well behaved or are not trained to stand quietly need a "corner" to restrict their movements. One possibility is to build a special room, based on the so-called "white room" of Bayer and Ehrlich (1965) and Ehrlich (1969) for standing human subjects (Fig. 5.9). Their room was 10 × 20 ft. and 10 ft. high, and the wall at one end merged into the floor with a cove of 5 ft. radius and into the ceiling with a 4 ft. radius. Everything in the room was painted "titanium flat white" except the floor of the traffic area, a 10 × 10 ft. area away from the coved end which was covered by light grey tiles. The light from an 800 joule electronic flash unit was bounced off the ceiling to produce a shadowless but directed diffuse lighting. This is similar in principle to the "all-white cubicle" lighting described for photographing bleached bones (see "Skeletal System"). Such a room could be modified for photography of animal patients by having an elevated bench coved to the wall and the wall-wall and wall-ceiling junctions coved at the site and the joints filled and sanded. A 3 ft. wide bench coved to the wall of a 12 ft.

wide room would give 4 ft. of flat bench and two coves of 4 ft. radius at each end, which should be sufficient to restrain most small animals for photography. Unfortunately, the color and tone of the wall would not be able to be changed, and thus a compromise would have to be made to select a background suitable for both color and monochrome photography. A light grey background of approximately 40 percent reflectance and thus lighter than a Kodak Neutral Test Card (18% reflectance) should be tried. "White rooms" are most suitable for monochrome prints, as white backgrounds are glaring in projected transparencies.

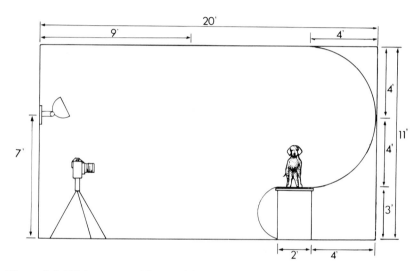

Figure 5.9. White room with coved background and bounce-flash illumination.

2. **Plain Concrete Wall and Apron.** The one described for large animals (Fig. 5.1) can also be used for small animals, particularly when abnormalities of gait are to be photographed. However, within the clinic itself, there are several alternative approaches. The basic requirement is for a plain light grey wall and floor with an unobtrusive wall-floor junction. Depending on the budget available, the options are (Gibson, 1948):

   a. Minimal Background. This can be a regular plain wall and floor. Paint the wall and baseboard light grey and install a floor covering such as sheet vinyl of the same color.
   b. Better Background. Remove the baseboard and caulk the wall-floor junction and have both the same light grey color as described in "a".
   c. Best Background. Cove the wall to the floor. It may be possible to

extend the sheet vinyl across the floor for 5 to 6 ft. and then up the wall for 4 to 6 ft. to provide a homogeneous light grey background. It would be even more desirable to have the background at the corner of the room, as this helps to restrain animals. The background walls should extend 6 to 8 ft. on the major wall and 3 to 5 ft. on the other wall.

If none of these alternatives are possible, then a pull-down paper background can be used.

3. **Pull-Down Backgrounds of Rolls of Paper Supported From the Wall or Ceiling.** These are commercially available. Paper is pulled down across the top of an ordinary 3 ft. high laboratory bench or examination table and over the front edge of the bench (Fritts, 1976) so that there are no sharp horizontal creases, only smooth curves (Figs. 5.10 and 5.11). Paper can also be pulled down the wall and over the floor, but the photographer will have to kneel. This arrangement may be more suitable for less cooperative and large, heavy dogs. Background paper over benches works for well-behaved small animals. It has the advantages that it can be located conveniently in or near examination or treatment rooms and occupies no space until it is pulled down. These backgrounds are similar to those recommended for large animals, except that the paper also covers the surface on which the animal stands. Because the rolls of paper need to be only 6–8 ft. wide, they are relatively cheap and rolls of different grey-toned paper can be installed. Thus, the tone of the grey background best suited for that subject can be selected, whether it is contrasting to emphasize the outline or a similar tone to be unobtrusive. It is an advantage to have the bench deeper than the usual 2 ft. A depth of 30 to 36 inches is recommended so that there is sufficient space between the subject and background to allow shadows cast from the lights mounted above the camera to fall onto the bench top rather than onto the background. The background roll of paper can be mounted behind an island bench and draped as in Figure 5.11. This has the advantage of allowing the background to be placed a few feet behind the subject. The photographer will need a minimum of 5–6 ft. of clear floor space adjacent to the bench, whether it is island or wall-mounted.

4. **Black from Background in Shadow.** This technique is similar to that used for photography of large animals where the subject is illuminated by the sun and the background is in shadow. However, in this case, lighting is from electronic flash and the animal stands on a table in an open doorway or in the middle of a large room so that the distance to the

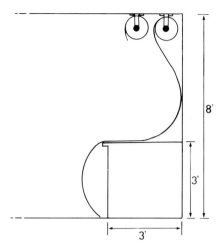

Figure 5.10. Small animal photographic background. Pull-down seamless background suspended from the ceiling and extending over the wall-mounted bench. The two rolls hold different backgrounds, e.g. light and dark grey.

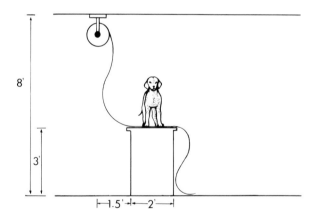

Figure 5.11. Small animal photographic background. Pull-down seamless background suspended from the ceiling and extending over an island bench.

background is very long. The resulting background is almost black, unless either gleaming stainless steel or glass in the background reflect specular highlights.

5. **Black Velvet.** Black velvet is superb for producing a full black background, even when directly illuminated. The deep black nap reflects only approximately 2%–3% of incident light. Black velvet can be used in the same way as paper backgrounds (Fig. 5.10). Striking photographs of

chickens with pendulous xanthomas and with curled-toe paralysis from vitamin B_2 deficiency have been made by using velvet background to emphasize the change in outline. Velvet must be kept clean because debris such as feathers, dander and feces are clearly visible. Lamoreaux (1941) minimized this problem by using a large piece of black velveteen as the background but placed an additional small piece to cover the surface upon which the bird stood. Good quality black velvet is expensive and its use should be reserved for use with clean small animals and birds where changes in outline need to be emphasized. Only disposable remnants of velvet should be used in the necropsy room.

6. **Pure White Backgrounds and Silhouettes.** These can be obtained by means of a transilluminated background. Kodak (1972a) described full-length (human) illuminators constructed with banks of fluorescent tubes behind a plastic panel. For smaller areas, they recommend an x-ray illuminator. The intensity of illumination from the background and on the subject should be balanced, as flare will result if the illuminator is too much brighter than the subject. The procedure is similar to that described under "Techniques to Obtain White Backgrounds."

For silhouettes, Kodak (1972a) recommends that:

    a. the intensity of the illuminator be read with a reflected light exposure meter.

    b. the illuminator be turned off and the subject lit to ¼ to ⅓ of the brightness of the illuminator.

    c. that portion of the illuminator outside the field of view of the camera be masked off to minimize flare.

White backgrounds and silhouettes are usually used only for monochrome prints, as a white background is too glaring in projected transparencies.

Lighting for Large and Small Animal Photography

The wisest procedure is to have clinical photographs of animals taken by a skilled photographer. If this is not possible, lighting and backgrounds should be designed in consultation with him. Lighting should be flexible to emphasize the lesion or clinical condition. Types of lighting include:

    1. Direct sunlight

    2. Diffused light from sky or overcast sky

    3. Available room light

4. Studio lights
5. Electronic flash

1. **Direct Sunlight.** Sunlight is an inflexible form of lighting. Its angle of illumination is fixed and may be unsuitable for photography at some times during the day. In the tropics, the sun is overhead and produces harsh contrasting shadows which require additional "fill-in" illumination. Even light reflected off the concrete apron and wall is inadequate to illuminate shadows. The color temperature of sunlight is approximately correct for daylight color films at noon when there is a mixture of direct sunlight and reflected skylight from clouds. The big disadvantage of daylight is that its color temperature varies with the time of the year, time of day and weather conditions (George, 1973). On perfectly cloud-less days, the illumination is bluish and produces a bluish-cast in transparencies. Sunlight can be used for rim lighting, but as a very low lighting angle is required, only very early or very late sunlight is suitable. However, an inevitable disadvantage is that transparencies have a yellowish or orange color cast, because sunlight, very early or late in the day, is low in color temperature.

If an outdoor concrete apron and wall are used as a background, the only way to adjust the angle of lighting is by positioning the subject. To have the flexibility to do this, a large background is required and hence we recommend a 60–100 ft. × 15 ft. high concrete wall. If the shadows are too dense, supplementary lighting is essential. This can be supplied by electronic flash. Cameras with focal plane shutters are at a disadvantage, because the fastest shutter speed synchronizing with electronic flash is usually 1/60 to 1/125 second. The other alternative is to use a studio light with a 5500°K bulb. This lamp can be positioned to give the desired degree of fill-in light to the shadows. Cameras with automatic exposure metering will insure reasonably correct exposure, but the light output of the fill-in lamp and its position should be planned by an experienced photographer. Usually, lights will be close to the camera's optical axis. The problem of selecting the correct exposure, when the intensity of sunlight fluctuates as clouds move across the face of the sun, has been solved by using modern automatic exposure cameras.

2. **Skylight or Overcast Sky.** Diffuse light from an overcast sky or one covered by light cloud is the best light source for outdoor photographs. Although the light is diffused, it is directional and produces a small degree of modeling. Color temperature is high and this results in a blue

color cast which can be corrected by light-balancing filters. They are probably not worth the time and trouble. This type of lighting is excellent for monochrome photographs, particularly if the negative is given additional development time (usually about 10%) to increase contrast. Most of these photographs will be of large animals. Small animals are better photographed indoors with artificial light which can be controlled.

3. **Available Room Light.** This is generally unsuitable because of its low level of illumination and incorrect color temperature. Even in well-lighted rooms with 100 ft. candles of illumination on the subject, exposures are 1/60 second at f-4 on 200 ISO transparency film. This is too slow to "freeze" subject movement and provide adequate depth of field. Thus, available room light can be used only for immobile subjects such as unconscious animals or cadavers.

4. **Studio Lamps.** High-output studio lamps are not used much in the photography of animals. Such equipment is expensive, requires the services of a skilled photographer, and the light and heat distract the animal's attention. Details of the lighting for a human clinical photographic studio have been described by Kodak (1972a).

5. **Electronic Flash.** This has major advantages for clinical photography. Exposures are so short (less than 1/1000 second) that any motion, either of the subject or the camera, is "frozen." Thus, cameras can be hand-held. Also, the light of electronic flash units has a color temperature of approximately 5500°K and is thus balanced for daylight color film. Over the years all sorts of combination of flash has been tried for the photography of animals: direct flash which produces harsh shadows, "bounce" flash from walls or umbrellas which produces soft diffuse light, and multiple flash units with "slave" units supplying fill-in illumination. Some units contain modeling lights so that the placement of the flash could be evaluated before the exposure was made. Many of these arrangements were excellent for studios but had severe limitations in photographing animals to illustrate lesions. One of these disadvantages was cost, but a major problem was the need to render texture and surface detail in skin lesions. For these, a main or texture light with a fill-in light was essential.

The same equipment recommended for cadaver photography and described under "Equipment" is highly suited for clinical photography of small animals. This unit consists of two matched dedicated flash units synchronized together and with the exposure controlled by the camera. The fill-in flash is mounted on the camera and operated at ¼ or ⅛ of the power of the main light. This can be done either by a selector switch on those flash units that have this feature or by covering the light by neutral density filters (LeBeau, 1985). Blaker (1977f) recommends that the main light be positioned 30° to 40° to the side and 30° to 40° above the camera's optical axis and pointing down at the subject. The flash may be held by the photographer if the subject is close, otherwise an assistant will be required to position the main light correctly. Usually, the main light will be to the left, but with clinical subjects it is more important that live animals face into the light so that the shadow is thrown behind the head. The fill-in flash is usually operated at 1/4 output, but if the (main light) flash-subject distance is larger than the camera-subject distance, it may be necessary to reduce the output of the fill-in flash to 1/8 to obtain a lighting ratio of 1:4 to 1:3.

For extreme close-up photography of skin, a different approach has to be taken because of the difficulty of accurately positioning the flash units. Basically, the same approach is used, but the flash units are mounted on a Lepp Macro-Rod (see "Equipment"). The rod is then screwed into the tripod bushing of the camera.

The use of electronic bounce flash units in a "white room" has been described above. Because "bounce" flash units do not direct all their light onto the subject, they have to have a higher output than flash units used to illuminate the subject directly. Thus, bounce units have to be more powerful and are consequently more expensive than those used for direct flash. Very high output units (e.g. 800–1000 joules) are required for whole body photographs of large animals, because the size of the subject to be illuminated and the long flash-subject distance control the intensity of illumination. The tendency is to keep this distance at a minimum so that a maximum amount of light is supplied to the subject, but a long subject-flash distance has the advantage of providing a more diffused, even illumination with less obvious shadows cast on the background.

Planning of Backgrounds for New Facilities

The objective of planning is to provide convenient and easily cleaned backgrounds which appear plain and unobtrusive in photographs. From the preceding discussion, it is obvious that the decisions to be made can be considered under four major categories: (1) clinical photographs of large animals; (2) clinical photographs of small animals; (3) photographs of live animals in a pathology laboratory or diagnostic laboratory; and (4) photographs of laboratory and zoo animals.

Large Animals. Here the major consideration has to be given to the decision whether or not to have a concrete wall and apron, preferably coved together either outside or inside the building or both. If a concrete wall would spoil the architectural beauty of the building because an unobtrusive site is not available or the wall cannot be screened, authorities may veto its construction. Of all of the backgrounds listed above, this is the most important and most desirable. It can be used not only for still photography of large and small animals but also for television and motion pictures of moving animals to show change in gait and posture. Without such a background, these photographs will still be taken but inevitably they will have distracting backgrounds.

Even if an outside wall with an apron is available, the second decision is whether or not to have an inside area for still photography. This area would be used in inclement weather or when outside lighting is unsuitable. In a large animal veterinary hospital there are usually several potential sites. These include large animal examination rooms, junctions of corridors at T-intersections and long wide corridors (Fig. 5.12). T-shaped studios have been recommended to save space in human hospitals (Gibson, 1948). The crossbar of the T is the patient area and the stem of the T provides the space to accommodate the working distance of the camera. Another possibility is the large animal examination room, many of which are 50 × 35 ft. with heights of 12 to 16 ft. With prior planning one wall could be kept plain, plastered and coved to the floor. This would be an excellent background. The height could be maintained at 16 ft. by placing pipes, air conditioning ducts and other impedimenta on another wall. Similarly, the drains for that floor should not be placed along the wall to be coved. In some veterinary hospitals, there are extremely long corridors of 100 to 150 ft. and usually about 16 ft. wide. The effective height in these varies from as high as 16 ft. to as low as 10 ft. if air conditioning ducts and lights are installed. Again, with advance planning the wall can be kept plain and pipes, ducts and drains positioned on the other side of the hallway.

Hallways offer two potential sites. One is at the junction of a T-shaped intersection and the other is along the length of the corridor. The latter will be useful only if the photographer has access through a door in the opposite wall so that a lens with sufficiently long working distance to prevent distortion can be used. Oblique views can be taken in a long corridor, but the background will not be as evenly illuminated as it would be on an outside wall illuminated by sun or skylight. If required,

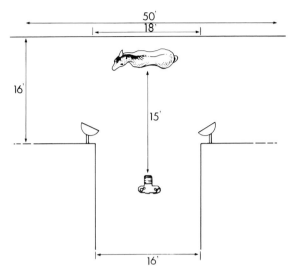

Figure 5.12. Plan of indoor large animal photographic background at junction of passageways in large animal veterinary hospital. The background is positioned at the intersection of passageways to allow a sufficiently long free-working distance for the camera.

permanently mounted flash units can be mounted high on the wall or ceiling.

Small Animals. The decisions are whether to have a special studio, pull-down backgrounds in examination and/or treatment rooms, a coved background built into one side of the treatment room or several of these options. Unless the studio is conveniently located, it may not be used. Certainly at least as a minimum, pull-down backgrounds should be planned for treatment rooms. These facilitate photography of sick animals. The only additional cost may be that incurred by strengthening the ceiling, for example, a suspended ceiling. Also, the position of the benches should be planned so that the photographer has sufficient room to move to photograph animals from different positions.

Veterinary Diagnostic Laboratories. If the diagnostic laboratory is in a veterinary school, backgrounds for large and small live animals may be available in the clinical departments. However, in a self-contained diagnostic laboratory these backgrounds need to be planned. Also, animals intended for euthanasia and necropsy because of an infectious disease may not be welcome in a clinical department. Consequently, there should be some facilities in or adjacent to the necropsy laboratory to photograph such animals. Rarely will there be enough *inside* room for photography of live large animals, but an adjacent outside wall may be suitable.

An inside background for small animals is highly desirable. A pull-down background is not so suitable for small farm animals as for well-trained companion animals. Farm animals need some type of built-in restraint, and one method of doing this is to build the bench described above under "Small Animals, Portrait Studio." This bench coved to the back wall and preferably to the side walls and ceiling would restrain small farm animals such as piglets and also birds, particularly if they were seriously ill. Such a bench and wall could be installed on one wall of the photography room adjacent to the necropsy room. This would have to be modified from the diagram in Figure 1.2 by extending the length of the room away from the door. Another alternative is to have the bench and background built onto one wall of the necropsy laboratory itself. Such a bench should be made of concrete or fiberglass to facilitate cleaning by hosing.

Other Animals. The requirements for a laboratory animal facility are similar to those for the necropsy laboratory. Laboratory animals are not trained and need some restraint. To restrain a rat, Horton (1940) devised a glass-sided enclosure which was 6 inches wide, 18 inches long and 12 inches high. The front and ends were glass and interchangeable. Clear glass, ground glass or colored backgrounds could be inserted. Lamoreaux (1941) found that "most domestic fowl can be persuaded to stand more or less naturally on a box or stand about 1 ft. square." The subject of photography of small laboratory animals has been reviewed by LeBeau (1987). He devised a rotatable pedestal stage consisting of a circular stage mounted on a vertical column supported on a 12 inch diameter base. The photographer could rotate the stage by turning the column. To be suitable for different-sized laboratory animals, three different stages (5, 8 and 15 inches diameter) and three columns (5, 8 and 12 inches high) were made. The circular stages were covered by a black velvet bootie. A similar pedestal, made from an 8 inch high can covered by snugly fitting black velveteen, had been described by Fritts (1976). However, LeBeau (1987) combined the pedestal stage with a "white room" or "white cubicle" 24 to 36 inches high and with a base approximately 24 inches square covered by white sailcloth (Fig. 5.13). A flash unit was placed in each front corner, at half the height of the cubicle and directed towards the opposite rear and upper corner, to provide diffused bounce light. A little of the light from the flash unit was deflected downward onto the subject by a reflector card on the flash unit. A black velvet background card just sufficiently large for each animal provided the black background. Some rabbits required a 14 × 14 inch card, but larger rabbits needed a 24 × 24 inch card. Exposure was determined by a flash meter, but adjustments in exposure had to be made because of the different reflectivity of the hair coats. Thus, for dark-haired guinea pigs, the aperature had to be opened 1 to 1½ stops and closed at ½ stop for white animals. LeBeau (1987) found that the repeatability of correct exposure was excellent and the photographer was able to adjust the animal's position within minutes using the rotatable stage. The lighting gave excellent rendition of the hair (Fig. 5.13).

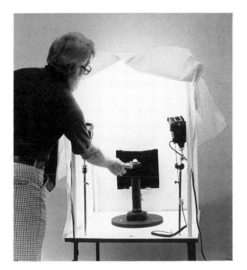 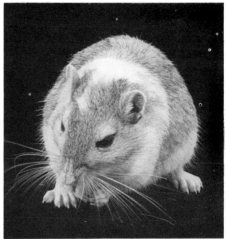

Figure 5.13. (*Left*) Rotatable background in a small "white room". (*Right*) Guinea pig photographed with black background in apparatus. Courtesy of Doctor L. J. LeBeau and *Journal of Biological Photography*.

Backgrounds for aquaria have been described by Gibson (1939, 1944) and Kodak (1972b). The problems of photography of aquaria including difficulties from the glass, clarity of water, reflections and backgrounds have been discussed in depth by George (1973). For zoo animals, a plain contrasting background is recommended by Dunton (1944). The outside wall and coved apron described above for large animals could be used but would need modification, for example, the height would have to be increased above 15 ft. to accommodate animals such as giraffes.

Summary

Adequate facilities for photography of live animals are minimal or even absent in many veterinary institutions. Photographic facilities should be designed when new buildings are planned. If included in the initial construction, plain concrete backgrounds and aprons, either outside or inside the building, are relatively inexpensive. At that time, walls can be planned to be plain without grills or utility services and finished in plain concrete without joints and with the wall-to-wall and wall-to-floor junctions coved. The cost to do this work later as a renovation may be prohibitive. If no backgrounds are available for live animals, the photographer is faced with making the best of what is available. For small animals, pull-down paper backgrounds are relatively inexpensive and easy to install. However, backgrounds for large animals are a problem. The solution usually becomes a matter of selecting the least objectionable background. Large expanses of concrete or asphalt can be checked to find a relatively homogeneous area, free of drains, for use as a background in photographs taken from a high viewpoint. An existing brick wall can be concreted and coved to eliminate vertical and horizontal lines (Fig. 5.4). Because daylight will be used for outside photographs, the times of day when illumination is suitable should be determined by observation. The large animal hospital may have an extensive inside area that can be modified to provide a plain background and floor. Lighting, usually electronic flash, can be installed suspended from the ceiling or wall so that the light comes from above and the units would be out of the way of horses and cleaning hoses. Finally, if no improvement can be made in the backgrounds of photographs of large animal(s), the services of an expert photographic retoucher should be used to eliminate disturbing backgrounds in prints for publication.

REFERENCES

American Society of Clinical Pathologists: Third annual 1981 medical photography competition. *Lab Med, 13*(2):122, 1982.

Anonymous: Photography of gross specimens—based on use of the Kodak precision enlarger. *Radiogr Clin Photogr, 18*(2):36–43, 1942.

Anonymous: Cutting the cord. *Popular Photography, 94*(4):134, 1987.

Armed Forces Institute of Pathology: *Manual of Macropathological Techniques.* Armed Forces Institute of Pathology, Medical Museum Laboratory, Washington, D.C., 1957.

Barnes, R. B., Burton, C. J., and Scott, R. G.: Electron microscopical replica techniques for the study of organic surfaces. *J Appl Physics, 16:*730–739, 1945.

Bayer, L. M., and Ehrlich, S.: Consistent shadowless photography in a growth research institute. *Med Radiogr Photogr, 41:*23–27, 1965.

Beiter, John J.: Blackened shields for clear lamps in medical photography. *J Biol Photogr Assoc, 15:*46–48, 1946.

Beiter, John J., and Bohrod, Milton G.: Transilluminated color backgrounds in medical photography. *J Biol Photogr Assoc, 13*(1):5–9, 1940.

Beiter, John J., Bohrod, Milton G., and Thomas, Harold A.: Control of highlights in the photography of gross specimens. *J Biol Photogr Assoc, 18:*67–74, 1950.

Blaker, A. A.: *Handbook for Scientific Photography.* San Francisco, Freeman, 1977a, pp. 39–46.

Blaker, A. A.: *Handbook for Scientific Photography.* San Francisco, Freeman, 1977b, pp. 47–68.

Blaker, A. A.: *Handbook for Scientific Photography.* San Francisco, Freeman, 1977c, p. 181.

Blaker, A. A.: *Handbook for Scientific Photography.* San Francisco, Freeman, 1977d, p. 189.

Blaker, A. A.: *Handbook for Scientific Photography.* San Francisco, Freeman, 1977e, pp. 193–194 and p. 254.

Blaker, A. A.: *Handbook for Scientific Photography.* San Francisco, Freeman, 1977f, pp. 210–213 and p. 256.

Bohrod, Milton G., and Beiter, John J.: Photography in color of fixed pathologic specimens. *J Lab Clin Med, 29:*994–997, 1944.

Brain, E. B.: Photographing specimens immersed in fluid. *Ann R Coll Surg Eng, 53*(3):194–196, 1973.

Breckenridge, Ella May Shackelford, and Halpert, Bela: The photography of gross specimens. *J Biol Photogr Assoc, 21:*1–14, 1953.

Bridgman, Charles F., and Humelbaugh, Frank A.: Plastic embedded teaching specimens. *Med Biol Illus, 13*(3):177–185, 1963.

Brown, David: Clean anatomical specimens. *Med Biol Illus, 8:*30–33, 1958.

Bullock, Gillian R., and Parson, Rodney R.: Photography in pharmacological research. In Newman, A. A. (Ed.): *Photographic Techniques in Scientific Research.* London, Academic Press, 1976, vol. II, pp. 1–42.

Burgess, Colin A.: Gross specimen photography—A survey of lighting and background techniques. *Med Biol Illus, 25:*159–166, 1975.

Burns, Steven T.: How to improve your clinical photography. *Mod Vet Pract, 60:*637, 1979.

Burry, A.F., and Stewart, B.: A simple method of eliminating highlights in photography of fresh specimens. *Med Biol Illus, 23:*55, 1973.

Callender, R.M.: The optical texture of human skin. *Med Biol Illus, 24*(4):172–173, 1974.

Carl, J.: Using a scale when photographing specimens. *Functional Photography, 15*(3):25–31, 1980.

Clarke, Carl D.: Apparatus for macrophotography. *J Biol Photogr Assoc, 2*(2):76–93, 1933.

Consumer Union: Glass cleaners, ratings. *Consumer Reports, 45*(9):570–571, 1980.

Daguid, Keith, and Ollerenshaw, Robert: Standardization in records of the foot. *Med Biol Illust, 12:*241–245, 1962.

Del Campo, C. H., Steffenhagen, W. P., and Ginther, O. J.: Clearing technique for preparation and photography of anatomic specimens of blood vessels of female genitalia. *Am J Vet Res, 35:*303–310, 1974.

Dent, R. V.: An infinitely variable background. *Brit J Photogr,* 709–710, 1937.

Dukes, Brian M.: Gross specimen photography. Mimeographed notes. Department of Pathology, Division of Medical Media Services, Western Pennsylvania Hospital, Pittsburgh, PA, 15224.

Dunton, S.C.: Certain problems in zoo photography. *J Biol Photogr Assoc, 13*(1):29–34, 1944.

Editors: How to do almost anything. *Modern Photog, 51*(1):15, 1987.

Ehrlich, S.: A white room for clinical photography. *Med Biol Illus, 19:*229–232, 1969.

Ellis, John: Under-fluid gross specimen photography—recent observations. *J Biol Photogr Assoc, 45:*98–99, 1977.

Emery, J. L., and Marshall, A. G.: *Handbook for Mortuary Technicians.* Oxford, Blackwell Scientific Publications, 1965.

Engel, C. E.: The department. In Linsen, E. F. (Ed.): *Medical Photography in Practice.* London, Fountain Press, 1961, pp. 22–23.

Fletcher, R. T.: Photography in ophthalmology. In Williams, Robin (Ed.): *Medical Photography Study Guide.* Lancaster, MTP Press Ltd., 1984, pp. 115–131.

Fox, Jay T.: Biological macrophotography with Kodachrome film. *J Biol Photogr Assoc, 11*(4):145–151, 1943.

Fritts, Donald H.: Basic veterinary field and clinical photography. In *Biomedical Photography: A Kodak Seminar.* Publication No. N-19, Rochester, Eastman Kodak, 1976, pp. 87–116.

Geddes, Nicholas: Adjustable scale-supports for specimen photography. *J Audiovis Media Med, 3*(4):142–144, 1980.

George, J. D.: Photography of living marine animals. In Cruise, J., and Newman, A. (Eds.): *Photographic Techniques in Scientific Research.* London, Academic Press, 1973, pp. 1–54.

Gibson, H. L.: Photography small live fish in full color. *J Biol Photogr Assoc, 8*(1):1–6, 1939.

Gibson, H. L.: Kodachrome photography of tropical fish in their own tank. *J Biol Photogr Assoc, 13*(2):65–72, 1944.

Gibson, H. L.: Planning the medical photographic department. *Med Radiogr Photogr, 24*(3):66–78, 1948.

Gibson, H. L.: Catch lights on gross specimens. *Med Radiogr Photogr, 25*(4):100–101, 1949.

Gibson, H. L.: Backgrounds for scientific photography—illustrated with reproductions from the 1949 exhibition of the biological photographic association. *Med Radiogr Photogr, 26*(3&4):118–121, 1950.

Gibson, H. L.: Lighting technics for medical photography. *Med Radiogr Photogr, 27*(3):90–96, 1951.

Gibson, H.L.: Technical considerations in photomacrography. *Med Biol Illus, 2:*247–257, 1952.

Gibson, H.L.: The Biological Photographic Association, its half century. *J Biol Photogr Assoc, 47*(2):82–96, 1979.

Gogolewski, R. P., Leathers C. W., Liggitt, H. D., and Corbeil, L. B.: Experimental Haemophilus somnus pneumonia in calves and immunoperoxidase localization of bacteria. *Vet Pathol,* 24:250–256, 1987.

Haber, Seth L.: Photography for the pathologist. *Lab World, 31*(9):16–19, 1980.

Haber, Seth L.: Photography for pathologists. *Pathologist, 36*(11):592–594, 1982.

Haber, Seth L.: Choosing a camera body. *Pathologist, 37*(5):339–341, 1983a.

Haber, Seth L.: Choosing a lens for your camera. *Pathologist, 37*(8):570–573, 1983b.

Haber, Seth L.: Choosing a film for your camera. *Pathologist, 38*(3):186–188, 1984.

Haeberlein, Charles: Specimen photography. In Hansell, Peter (Ed.): *A Guide to Medical Photography.* Baltimore, University Park Press, 1979, pp. 77–97.

Halsman, Julius: Standards in gross photography. *J Biol Photogr Assoc, 23*(2&3):119–125, 1955.

Halsman, J., and Ishak, K. G.: Photography and medical illustration. In Race, G. J. (Ed.): *Laboratory Medicine.* Hagerstown, Harper and Row, 1977, vol. 3, pp. 1–15.

Hampton, R., and Clarke, N. M. P.: A guide to the photography of cleared small bone specimens. *J Biol Photogr, 51*(3):85–87, 1983.

Hansell, Peter: Medical photography—a review. *Lancet, 251:*296–299, 1946.

Hansell, Peter: Some observations on dermatological photography. *J Biol Photogr Assoc, 16:*51–55, 1947.

Hansell, Peter: Letters to the editor. *J Biol Photog, 53*(2):41, 1985.

Hansell, Peter, and Ollerenshaw, Robert: Design of the department. In *Longmore's Medical Photography,* 7th ed. Philadelphia, Lippincott, 1962, pp. 209–222.

Hansell, Peter, and Ollerenshaw, Robert: Background. *Longmore's Medical Photography,* 7th ed. Philadelphia, Lippincott, 1962, pp. 200–206.

Hansell, Peter, and Ollerenshaw, Robert: Photography of gross specimens. *Longmore's Medical Photography,* 7th ed. Philadelphia, Lippincott, 1962, pp. 329–353.

Hansell, Peter, and Ollerenshaw, Robert: Photography of the skin. *Longmore's Medical Photography,* 7th ed. Philadelphia, Lippincott, 1962, pp. 288–290.

Harp, David H.: Adjustable scale stand for gross specimen photography. *J Biol Photogr Assoc, 33:*(3)125–127, 1965.

Harris, Stanley D.: Background brilliance in gross-specimen photography. *Med Radiogr Photogr, 32:*(1)21–23, 1956.

Harrison, Norman K.: Photographing pathological specimens. *Functional Photography,* London, *1:*22–23, 1950.

Harrison, Norman K.: Equipment for medical photography. In Linssen, E. F. (Ed.): *Medical Photography in Practice.* London, Fountain Press, 1961, pp. 319–322.

Heard, B. E., and Brackenbury, W.: Demonstration of pulmonary emphysema. *Med Biol Illus, 12*(2):112.

Horton, Nathan S.: Some notes on photography of the albino rat. *J Biol Photogr Assoc, 9*(1):5–9, 1940.

Hund, Dietmar: The photography of patients. In Hansell, Peter (Ed.): *A Guide to Medical Photography.* Baltimore, University Park Press, 1979, pp. 9–15.

Hurtgen, Thomas P.: Kodak color films for medical photography. *Med Radiogr Photogr 54*(2):22–30, 1978.

Jenny, L., and Panozzo-Heilbronner, R.: Problems in practical macrography and incident-light micrography. Part 2: Arrangement and presentation of the subject. *Microskopion, 38:*4–12, 1981.

Kennedy, Lloyd A.: Techniques for photography of immersed specimens. *J Biol Photog, 52*(3):67–74, 1984.

Kennedy, Lloyd A.: Letters to the editor. *J Biol Photog, 53*(2):41, 1985.

Kennedy, Lloyd A.: A traction apparatus for specimen photography. *J Biol Photogr, 54*(3):85–87, 1986.

Kent, F. W.: Medical photography in a teaching hospital. *Med Radiogr Photogr, 23*(1):13–36, 1947.

Kent, F. W.: This issue's cover subject. *Med Radiogr Photogr, 24*(3):cover and contents page, 1948.

Keppler, H.: Can an inexpensive zoom equal a touted micro lens? *Modern Photog, 49*(8):40–41, 118, 120, 1985.

Klotz, Oskar: The staining of pathological specimens in the gross. *Bull Int Assoc Med Museums, 5:*51–53, 1915.

Klotz, Oskar, and Maclachlan, W. W. G.: A modified Jores' method for the preservation of colors in gross specimens. *Bull Int Assoc Med Museums, 5:*59–60, 1915.

Kodak: *The Photography of Gross Specimens.* Kodak publication N-5, Revised ed., Rochester, Eastman Kodak, 1966.

Kodak: *Basic Scientific Photography.* Kodak publication N-9, Rochester, Eastman Kodak, 1970.

Kodak: *Composition.* Kodak publication AC-11, Rochester, Eastman Kodak, 1971.

Kodak: *Clinical Photography.* Kodak publication N-3, Rochester, Eastman Kodak, 1972a.

Kodak: *Close-up Photography.* Kodak publication N-12A, Rochester, Eastman Kodak, 1972b.

Kodak: *Color as Seen and Photographed.* Kodak publication E-74H, 2nd ed., Rochester, Eastman Kodak, 1972c.

Kodak: *Small Lens Openings Destroy Image Sharpness.* Kodak publication Q-1104, Rochester, Eastman Kodak, 1978.

Kodak: *Reciprocity Data: Kodak Professional Filming.* Kodak publication E-31, Rochester, Eastman Kodak, 1983.

Kodak: Guides for identical tests when exposing color films with fluorescent or high-intensity discharge lamps. *Kodak Tech Bits.* Kodak publication P-3-84-3, Rochester, Eastman Kodak, 1984a, pp. 8–9.

Kodak: *Kodak Professional Black-and-White Films.* Kodak publication F-5, Rochester, Eastman Kodak, 1984b.

Kutscher, H.: Die photographische Dokumentation in der Dermatologie. *Der Deutsche Dermatologe, 31*(9):1174–1185, 1983.

Kutscher, Hans: Objectification of dermatological findings by photographic documentation. *Zeiss Information, 23*(86):20–23, 1978.

Lamoreaux, W. F.: Photographing domestic birds. *J Biol Photogr Assoc, 9*(4):195–199, 1941.

Laurence, K. M., and Martin, D.: A technique for obtaining undistorted specimens of the central nervous system. *J Clin Path, 12:*188–190, 1959.

LaBossiere, E.: *Histological Processing for the Neural Sciences.* Springfield, Charles C Thomas, 1976, p. 85.

Leapley, McK. A.: Gross specimen photo cabinet. *J Biol Photogr Assoc, 37*(2):112–114, 1969.

LeBeau, Leon J.: Control of infectious hazards for the biophotographer. *J Biol Photogr Assoc, 41*(4):96–100, 1973.

LeBeau, Leon J.: Versatile and compact stage for photographing small laboratory subjects. *J Biol Photogr Assoc, 48:*3–13, 1980.

LeBeau, Leon J., and Wimmer, A. D.: Photography of tiny reflective biomedical objects. *J Biol Photogr, 50*(4):101–120, 1982.

LeBeau, Leon J.: Evaluation of the medical-dental-bio-macro-bracket for small object photography. *J Biol Photogr, 53*(1):79–89, 1985.

LeBeau, Leon J., Pederson, E. K., Parshall, R. F., and Beluhan, F. Z.: Photography of small laboratory animals. Part two: techniques and procedures. *J Biol Photogr, 55*(3):99–105, 1987.

Levin, A.: Photographing gross specimens on Kodachrome film. *J Biol Photogr Assoc, 7*(3):113–115, 1939.

Lewin, Klaus, and Morton, Richard: The preservation of human tissues in a fresh state. *Med Biol Illus, 13*(3):159, 1963.

Lie, J. T.: Heart and vascular system. In Ludwig, J. (Ed.): *Current Methods of Autopsy Practice,* 2nd ed. Philadelphia, Saunders, 1979, Chapt. 3, pp. 21–50.

Loomis, Steven D.: A simple method of adding half-stops to a Micro Nikkor lens. *J Biol Photog, 52*(3):53–55, 1984.

Ludwig, J.: Tracheobronchial tree and lungs. In Ludwig, J. (Ed.): *Current Methods of Autopsy Practice,* 2nd ed. Philadelphia, Saunders, 1979a, Chapt. 4, pp. 51–74.

Ludwig, J.: Esophagus and abdominal viscera. In Ludwig, J. (Ed.): *Current Methods of Autopsy Practice,* 2nd ed. Philadelphia, Saunders, 1979b, Chapt. 5, pp. 75–94.

Ludwig, J.: Skeletal system. In Ludwig, J. (Ed.): *Current Methods of Autopsy Practice,* 2nd ed. Philadelphia, Saunders, 1979c, Chapt. 7, pp. 130–137.

Ludwig, J.: Autopsy laboratory procedures. In Ludwig, J. (Ed.): *Current Methods of Autopsy Practice,* 2nd ed. Philadelphia, Saunders, 1979d, Chapt. 9, p. 174.

Mallory, F. B., and Wright, J. M.: *Pathological Technique,* 7th ed. Philadelphia, Saunders, 1918.

Markson, L. M., and Wells, G. A. H.: Evaluation of autofluorescence as an aid to diagnosis of cerebrocortical necrosis. *Vet Rec, 111:*338–340.

Marshall, Ralph: Photographic background control. *Med Biol Illus, 7:*13–21, 1957.

Marshall, R. J., and Marshall, B. M.: Routine medical photography with 35 mm black-and-white film. *Med Biol Illus, 25:*115–119, 1975.

Martin, Derek: Care of specimens for illustration. *Med Biol Illus, 3:*216–223, 1953.

Martin, Derek: Gross pathological specimens. In Linssen, E. F. (Ed.): *Medical Photography in Practice.* London, Fountain Press, 1961, pp. 247–274.

Martinsen, William L. M.: Gross specimen photography—a review. *Med Biol Illus, 2:*179–191, 1952.

Martinsen, William L. M.: Photography of specimens. In Engel, C. E. (Ed.): *Photography for the Scientist.* London, Academic Press, 1968, pp. 451–480.

McGavin, M. D.: A technique for photographing the living bovine eye. *Aust Vet J, 37:*416–420, 1961a.

McGavin, M. D.: Simplified photography of gross pathological specimens. *Aust Vet J, 37:*443–450, 1961b.

McGavin, M. D., and Morrill, J. L.: Dissection technique for examination of the bovine ruminoreticulum. *J Anim Sci, 42*(2):535–538, 1976.

McGavin, M. D.: A suitable camera stand for macrophotography of pathological specimens. *Functional Photography, 17:*14–35, 1982.

Meiller, Fred H.: A method for preserving gross specimens in color. *J Techn Meth (Bull Internat Assoc Med Museums), 18:*57–58, 1938.

Mineo, Joseph: Reflection control in small object photography. *J Biol Photogr Assoc, 34*(3):101–106, 1966.

Morgan, W. D., and Lester, H. M.: *Leica Manual and Data Book,* 13th ed. London, Fountain Press, 1956, p. 408.

Mutter, E.: *Leica Fotografie,* (English Edition), (5):211–215, 1957.

Nickey, W. M., Dill, Russell, E., and Vendrell, Doris D.: Autopsy pathology and neuropathology. In Race, G. J. (Ed.): *Laboratory Medicine.* Hagerstown, Harper & Row, 1977, vol. 3, pp. 1–27.

Nippon Kogaku: *Micro-Nikkor Auto 55mm f3.5 Instructions.* Tokyo, Nippon Kogaku, K.K., 1969.

Okazaki, H., and Campbell, R. J.: Nervous system. In Ludwig, J. (Ed.): *Cur-*

rent *Methods of Autopsy Practice,* 2nd ed. Philadelphia, Saunders, 1979, pp. 95–129.

Olsen, E. G. J.: *The Pathology of the Heart.* New York, Intercontinental, 1973, p. 2.

Opps, Francis A.: A new camera box for the photography of gross pathological specimens. *J Biol Photogr Assoc, 2*(3):151–156, 1934.

Palgilinan, L.: Neonatal neuropathology dissection. *Res Staff Phys, 20*(28), 1974.

Paulson, Robert C.: Scales for scientific pictures. *Photogr App Sci Tech Med, 6:*16–18, 1971.

Pilcher, John F.: Autopsy room photography. *J Biol Photogr Assoc, 6:*61–64, 1937.

Pontiac Motor Division: *1986 Pontiac 6000 Owner's Manual.* Pontiac, Michigan, 1986.

Potter, A. R., and Evans, T. E. M.: A simple unit for specimen photography. *Forensic Photography, 3:*2–3, 1974.

Pulvertaft, R. J. V.: Museum techniques: A review. *J Clin Path, 3:*1–23, 1950.

Reiner, L.: Gross examination of the heart. In Gould, S. F. (Ed.): *Pathology of the Heart and Blood Vessels,* 3rd ed. Springfield, Charles C Thomas, 1968, pp. 1111–1149.

Rhea, L. J.: Field maceration. *Bull Internat Assoc Med Museums, 8:*40, 1922.

Robertson, S. J.: Photography in dermatology. In Williams, Robin (Ed.): *Medical Photography Study Guide.* Lancaster, MTP Press Ltd., 1984, pp. 89–100.

Rochow, Theodore George, and Rochow, Eugene George: *An Introduction to Microscopy by Means of Light, Electrons, X-rays, or Ultrasound.* New York, Plenum Press, 1978.

Rogers, George W.: Photography in paediatrics. In Newman, A. A. (Ed.): *Photographic Techniques in Scientific Research, 2:*142–231, 1976.

Rosenthal, S. E.: Rapid maceration technique for demonstrating the trabecular pattern in bones. *Bull Internat Assoc Med Museums, 28:*174–178, 1948.

Sacco, W. K.: Graphic presentation. *Functional Photography, 17*(4):17–31, 1982.

Salthouse, T. N.: The photography of gross specimens with fluorescent lighting. *Med Biol Illus, 5:*75–84, 1955.

Salthouse, T. N.: Photography of the negro skin. *Med Biol Illus, 8:*150–159, 1958.

Schaelow, Ernst: Transillumination in biological photography. *Med Biol Illus, 5:*143–146, 1955.

Schmidt, L., and Haulenbeek, J. B.: A method of photographing gross specimens. *J Biol Photogr Assoc, 1*(2):76–79, 1932.

Schummer, A., Nickel, R., and Sack, W. O.: *The Viscera of the Domestic Mammals,* 2nd rev. ed. Berlin, Parey, 1979.

Shaw, John. *The Nature Photographer's Complete Guide to Professional Field Techniques.* New York, Amphoto, 1984.

Shein, Melvin: Color restoration and preservation of gross museum specimens. *Bull Internat Assoc Med Museums, 32:*117–122, 1951.

Smialowski, Arthur, and Currie, Donald J.: Simplified photography of gross specimens using "S–C" photographic arrangement. *J Biol Photogr Assoc, 26*(3):115–119, 1958.

Smialowski, Arthur, and Currie, Donald J.: Gross specimen and cadaver photography. In *Photography in Medicine.* Springfield, Charles C Thomas, 1960a, Chapt. VII, pp. 83–104.

Smialowski, Arthur, and Currie, Donald J.: Photography in dermatology. In

Photography in Medicine. Springfield, Charles C Thomas, 1960b, Chapt. XI, pp. 158–165.

Smialowski, Arthur, and Currie, Donald J.: Surgical operating room still photography. *J Biol Photogr Assoc, 32*(4):150–160, 1964.

Smith, H. A., and Jones, T. C.: *Veterinary Pathology,* 2nd ed. Philadelphia, Lea & Febiger, 1961, p. 183.

Stanford, B.: The hospital photographic department. *Lancet, 251:*299–301, 1946.

Stenstrom, William J.: Photographing the external eye. *J Biol Photogr Assoc, 43*(2):70–73, 1975.

Stenstrom, William J.: Guidelines for external eye photography. *J Biol Photogr Assoc, 46*(4):155–158, 1978.

Tredinnick, D.: Photography in the pathologies. In Williams, Robin (Ed.): *Medical Photography Study Guide.* Lancaster, MTP Press Ltd., 1984, pp. 185–194.

Vetter, John P.: An integrated method of preserving and photographing gross specimens. *J Biol Photogr Assoc, 28*(1):21–34, 1960.

Vetter, John P.: Photographing gross specimens. *Lab Management, 7:*24–44, 1969.

Vetter, John P.: The color photography of gross specimens. *Pathologist, 38*(3):155–162, 1984.

Wagner, G., and Nuckolos, H. H.: Comparative study of various techniques for preparation of bone specimens for museum preparation. *Bull Internat Assoc Med Museums, 14:*35, 1936.

Walter, Ken: Universal x-ray copying and macro bench. *Med Biol Illus, 23:*217–220, 1973.

White, H.: Clinical photography in dermatologic office practice. *Cutis, 6*(10):1099–1103, 1970.

Whitley, Robert J.: In Linssen, E. F. (Ed.): *Medical Photography in Orthopaedic Surgery in Medical Photography in Practice.* London, Fountain Press, 1961, pp. 228–238.

Whitley, Robert J.: A versatile illuminator. *Med Biol Illus, 3:*39, 1953.

Williams, A. R.: In Morton, R. A. (Ed.): *Photography for the Scientist.* London, Academic Press, 1984, pp. 355–391.

Williams, Daniel C., and Roth, L. Evans: In Swenson, Melvin J. (Ed.): *Dukes Physiology of Domestic Animals,* 9th ed. Ithaca, Comstock, 1977, p. 38.

Winburne, L. D.: Photography of selected gross pathologic specimens under fluid. *J Biol Photogr Assoc, 25*(3):112–113, 1957.

Wolfe, G. Suitable stand for the photographing of pathological specimens. *Functional Photography, 18*(1):41, 1983.

Zorer, Wolfgang, and Deasy, Kevin: Simplified specimen photography. Standardized technique yields high-quality photos while saving time. *Biomed Commun, 10*(4):10–11, 1982.

INDEX